Liver Revival

Rejuvenate the Body's Detox Powerhouse

Liver Revival
Rejuvenate the Body's Detox Powerhouse

Copyright © *Levitas One*, 2024

All Rights Reserved

This book is subject to the condition that no part of this book is to be reproduced, transmitted in any form or means; electronic or mechanical, stored in a retrieval system, photocopied, recorded, scanned, or otherwise. Any of these actions require the proper written permission of the author.

What are the NoMAD Plans?

Developed by Dr Ash Kapoor, the NoMAD Plans represent a transformative approach to health and wellness that combines the wisdom of ancestral practices with contemporary medical insights. The name "NoMAD" not only suggests a journey through the intricate realm of health but also stands for its foundational principles: Nutritional Optimisation, Mindful Adaptation, and Detoxification.

At the heart of NoMAD is the 6R Framework—Restore, Release, Repair, Renew, Reframe, and Represent. This methodology addresses the root causes of illness, combats chronic inflammation, and cultivates authentic vitality, guiding individuals through a transformative process.

Tailored specifically to each individual, NoMAD journeys are meticulously crafted to rebalance the body, strengthen the mind, and rejuvenate overall health. By integrating ancestral practices with cutting-edge, innovative treatments—all under strict medical oversight—NoMAD Plans offer a personalised pathway to sustainable, long-lasting well-being that resonates with your unique life circumstances.

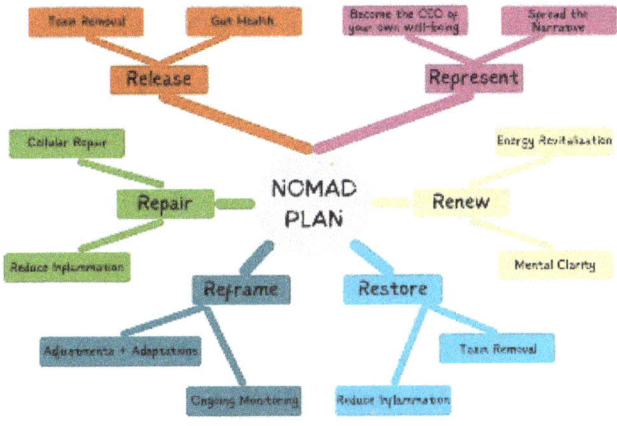

Levitas One:
"As Is In, As Is Out"

Reflecting the belief that our internal well-being is mirrored in our external environment. Founded by Dr. Ash Kapoor, Levitas One serves as the vehicle for delivering NoMAD's treatment plans. It envisions a healthcare future where patients are at the centre of a fully integrated, multidisciplinary approach. Guided by Nomads 6 Rs—Restore, Release, Repair, Renew, and Reframe, Represent—Levitas One empowers self-care through personalised guidance and minimal intervention, promoting long-term health, balance, and sustainability.

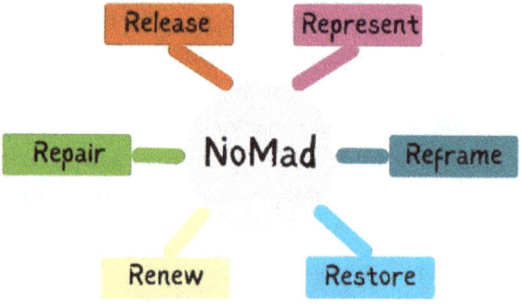

Contents

Preface viii

Chapter 1 Introduction to Liver Health and Detoxification 1
Overview of Liver Function 1
Detoxification Processes in the Liver 2
Common Signs of a Stressed Liver 3
Introduction to Liver-Related Diseases 4
Case History: A Middle-Aged Professional with a Stressed Liver 5
Conclusion 6
Summary: Introduction to Liver Health and Detoxification 6

Chapter 2 The Science Behind Liver Detox 7
Toxins and Liver Health 7
The Role of Inflammation 8
How Liver Detox Works 9
Lifestyle Factors that Impact Liver Detox 10
How to Support Liver Detox 11
Case History: Managing Inflammation with Liver Detox 12
Conclusion 13
Summary: The Science Behind Liver Detox 14

Chapter 3 Pharmacological Approaches to Liver Detox 15
Prescription Medications for Liver Health 15
TUDCA: A Bile Acid for Liver Detox 16
Medications for Heavy Metal Detox 18
Risks and Side Effects 19
Supporting Liver Health with Lifestyle Changes 20
Case History: Alcohol-Induced Liver Damage and Pharmacological Support 21
Conclusion 22
Summary: Pharmacological Approaches to Liver Detox 23

Chapter 4 Micronutrients for Liver Health 24
The Role of Micronutrients in Liver Detoxification 24
Key Micronutrients for Liver Health 25
Food Sources vs. Supplements 28
Micronutrient Deficiencies and Liver Disease 29
Case History: Micronutrient Deficiency and Liver Health 29
Conclusion 30
Chapter Summary: 31
Summary: Micronutrients for Liver Health 31

Chapter 5 Herbal and Botanical Support for Liver Detox 32
Popular Herbs for Liver Detox 32
Traditional Use vs. Modern Science 37
Case History: Herbal Detox Success Story 37
Incorporating Herbs into Your Liver Detox Routine 38
Safety Considerations When Using Herbs 39
Conclusion 40
Chapter Summary 40
Summary: Herbal and Botanical Support for Liver Detox 41

Chapter 6 The Role of Diet in Liver Detox 42
The Liver's Relationship with Food 42
Anti-Inflammatory Foods for Liver Health 42
Healthy Fats and Liver Detox 44
Foods to Avoid for Liver Health 45
Case History: Diet and Liver Detox Success Story 48
Conclusion 49
Chapter Summary 49
Summary: The Role of Diet in Liver Detox 50

Chapter 7 Fasting and Detoxification: A Powerful Strategy for Liver Health 51
How Fasting Benefits the Liver 51
Enhancing Fasting with Glutathione, NAC, and Deliverance 52
Fasting Methods for Liver Detox: A Positive Approach 54
Case History: Fasting with Glutathione, NAC, and Deliverance 55
Conclusion 56
Chapter Summary 56
Summary: Fasting and Detoxification: A Powerful Strategy for Liver Health 57

Chapter 8 IV Therapies and Light Therapy for Liver Detox 58
IV Therapies for Liver Detox 58
Scientific Backing for IV and Light Therapy 63
Case History: Liver Detox with IV Therapy and Light Therapy 64
Conclusion 64
Summary: IV Therapies and Light Therapy for Liver Detox 65

Chapter 9 Heavy Metal Toxicity and Detoxification 66
How Heavy Metals Impact the Liver 66
Symptoms of Heavy Metal Toxicity 67
Oligoscan Testing for Heavy Metal Toxicity 68
Strategies for Heavy Metal Detoxification 69
Case History: Detoxing from Mercury Exposure 71
Conclusion 72
Summary: Heavy Metal Toxicity and Detoxification 73

Chapter 10 Liver Detox for Children 74
Why Children Need Liver Detox Support 74
Safe Detox Solutions for Children 76
Detox Practices for Children...78
Case History: Liver Detox in a Child with Eczema 79
Conclusion 79
Chapter Summary..80
Summary: Liver Detox for Children 81

Chapter 11 Ancient Practices in Liver Health....................................... 82
Traditional Chinese Medicine (TCM) and Liver Detox 82
Ayurveda and Liver Health...84
The Liver and Pitta Dosha...84
Ancient Greek Medicine and the Liver...85
Modern Science Meets Ancient Wisdom 86
Conclusion 87
Chapter Summary..87
Summary: Ancient Practices in Liver Health 88

Glossary.. 89
References 93

Preface

Throughout my journey in regenerative medicine, I began to truly appreciate the profound role of the liver in detoxification. As clinicians, we are well-versed in the concept of **first-pass liver metabolism** when it comes to drugs and how the liver filters out substances before they enter the systemic circulation. However, I had not fully grasped the extent of the toxins that the liver contends with daily, especially in light of the modern environmental landscape.

We live in an era where we are constantly bombarded by pollutants—whether it is from the air we breathe, the water we drink, or the food we consume. These toxins accumulate, placing an overwhelming burden on the liver, which tirelessly works to filter and neutralise these harmful substances. This book delves into the staggering impact of environmental toxins on liver health and offers strategies to support and protect this vital organ.

One crucial realisation in my exploration was the interconnectedness between liver function and the gut—our **primary immune barrier**. When the gut is compromised, toxins more readily enter the bloodstream, placing an even greater burden on the liver. The rising incidence of gut issues, including **leaky gut syndrome** and dysbiosis, only exacerbates this problem, turning the liver into the body's overworked "doorman" trying to manage a flood of invaders.

In this book, I hope to provide you with insights into mitigating the risks linked to an overwhelmed liver, as well as the practical tools to fortify your body's natural detoxification systems. By focusing not just on liver health but also on **gut integrity**, you'll learn how to reduce toxin overload and protect your body's natural defences. The liver is not just a detoxifier—it is a silent guardian of our health, and it is time we give it the care and support it deserves.

With these pages, I invite you to join me in understanding the vital role of liver detoxification, the immense impact of our environment on our health, and the powerful ways we can protect the "doorman" of our bodies, ensuring it continues to function optimally for years to come.

— ***Ash Kapoor***

Chapter 1
Introduction to Liver Health and Detoxification

Overview of Liver Function

Imagine the liver as your body's own version of a high-tech waste management system combined with a multi-purpose processing plant. It has two major jobs: getting rid of harmful substances (toxins) and making sure your body gets the nutrients it needs from food. Without the liver working properly, your body would be overwhelmed with toxins, much like a city drowning in its own garbage if the waste collectors went on strike.

- **Detoxification:**

One of the liver's most important jobs is filtering toxins out of the blood. Every day, the liver breaks down chemicals from food, alcohol, medications, and pollutants, converting them into safer substances or packaging them up for elimination. It processes **1.4 litres of blood every minute**, meaning that the liver is constantly "cleaning" your bloodstream. If toxins are allowed to accumulate, they can cause damage to your brain, heart, and other organs. In a way, you can think of the liver as the body's built-in water filter—it catches the bad stuff and makes sure only clean, nutrient-rich blood circulates through your system.

- **Metabolism:**

The liver is also responsible for processing nutrients from the food you eat. It breaks down **carbohydrates** into glucose (sugar). It stores the glucose as **glycogen**, which acts as a quick source of energy when needed. If you skip a meal, the liver will release glucose to keep your blood sugar stable, ensuring your brain and muscles have enough fuel to function. Think of the liver like your body's energy warehouse—it stores and distributes energy based on demand.

- **Nutrient Storage and Bile Production:**

The liver also stores vitamins and minerals, like **vitamins A, D**, and **B12**. It produces **bile**, which is essential for digesting fats. Bile acts like dish soap in your digestive system, breaking down fat into smaller droplets so they can be absorbed by the intestines.

Detoxification Processes in the Liver

The liver's detoxification system can be broken down into two phases, which work together like a two-step cleaning process.

- **Phase 1: Oxidation**

In Phase 1, enzymes (primarily the **cytochrome P450** family) act like tiny workers, breaking down toxins into more reactive, often more harmful, substances. It is similar to a mechanic removing parts from a damaged car to expose the engine. What's left behind may still be toxic but is easier to deal with in the next step. Substances like **alcohol**, **caffeine**, and **medications** are processed in this stage.

However, this process also produces free radicals, which are like sparks flying off an engine—it is a natural part of the breakdown process but can cause damage if not managed. Without enough antioxidants like **vitamin C, E**, and **glutathione** to neutralise these free radicals, oxidative stress can occur, damaging the liver cells.

- **Phase 2: Conjugation**

This is where the liver adds molecules (like **glutathione, sulfate**, or **glycine**) to the reactive substances from Phase 1, making them water-soluble so they can be flushed out of the body via urine or bile. It is like taking the car parts that have been dismantled in Phase 1 and packaging them up to be safely discarded. Phase 2 is primarily dependent on sufficient nutrient intake, particularly antioxidants and amino acids from protein.

Common Signs of a Stressed Liver

Much like a factory that's running overtime, when the liver is overwhelmed, it sends out signals that it needs help. The problem is many of these signs are subtle and can be easily overlooked or misattributed to other health issues. Let us explore some of the most common signs of liver overload:

1. **Fatigue**:

    Feeling constantly tired, even after a good night's sleep? The liver might be struggling to keep up with detoxing your body, leading to a buildup of toxins that sap your energy. Imagine trying to run your car with a clogged air filter—it does not perform as well, and over time, it starts to stall. Similarly, a tired liver can make you feel sluggish and lethargic.

2. **Digestive Issues**:

    The liver plays a crucial role in digestion by producing bile, which helps break down fats. If your liver is stressed, bile production may drop, leading to bloating, gas, or even discomfort after eating fatty meals. If you frequently feel like your digestive system is off balance, it may be time to give your liver some attention.

3. **Skin Conditions**:

    Breakouts, rashes, or dry, irritated skin can be a sign that your liver is overwhelmed. When the liver can't keep up with detoxifying the body, toxins sometimes try to escape through the skin, leading to inflammation and irritation. Think of the skin as your body's backup detox organ—when the liver can't do its job, the skin steps in to help.

4. **Cognitive Fog**:

    If toxins build up in the blood due to poor liver function, they can affect brain function, leading to **brain fog**, memory issues, or trouble concentrating. Similar to how poor air quality can make it hard to breathe, a toxic internal environment makes it difficult for your brain to function at its best.

Introduction to Liver-Related Diseases

When the liver is under constant stress, it can lead to more severe health conditions. Let us look at a few critical liver-related diseases:

- **Non-Alcoholic Fatty Liver Disease (NAFLD):**

    This condition occurs when excess fat builds up in the liver, even if you don't drink alcohol. It is one of the most common liver disorders and is often linked to obesity, poor diet, and metabolic syndrome. Left untreated, NAFLD can progress to **non-alcoholic steatohepatitis (NASH)**, liver scarring (**fibrosis**), and eventually **cirrhosis**.

- **Hepatitis:**

    This is inflammation of the liver, often caused by viral infections (Hepatitis A, B, or C), but it can also result from toxin exposure, excessive alcohol use, or autoimmune reactions. Inflammation is like a constant state of "red alert" in the liver—over time, this can lead to permanent damage.

- **Cirrhosis:**

    Think of cirrhosis as the liver's version of a scar. It happens after long-term damage from inflammation or toxins. The liver tissue becomes fibrotic, reducing its ability to perform its functions. Cirrhosis is irreversible and often leads to liver failure if not managed early.

Liver Revival

Case History: A Middle-Aged Professional with a Stressed Liver

Background:

Mark, a 45-year-old marketing executive, had a diet high in processed foods and was a regular social drinker. He spent most of his days sitting at his desk, and although he didn't feel "sick," he often complained of feeling tired, bloated, and stressed. His skin was prone to breakouts, and he noticed that he had difficulty concentrating, especially after lunch.

The Issue:

After a routine blood test revealed elevated liver enzymes (**ALT** and **AST**), his doctor suggested that his liver was under stress. These enzymes are markers of liver damage and can indicate conditions like **NAFLD** or early-stage liver inflammation.

Detox Plan:

Mark's detox plan was simple but effective:

1. **Dietary Changes**: He eliminated processed foods, added more fresh vegetables and lean proteins, and reduced his alcohol intake. Leafy greens, which boost bile production, became a staple in his meals.

2. **Herbal Supplements**: Mark started taking **milk thistle** and **turmeric**, both known for their liver-supporting properties.

3. **Exercise and Hydration**: He introduced a daily walk into his routine and increased his water intake to help flush out toxins.

Results:

After six months, Mark's liver enzyme levels returned to normal, and he reported feeling more energised. His digestive issues resolved, and he noticed fewer breakouts on his skin. The simple changes allowed his liver to catch up and detoxify more efficiently.

Conclusion

The liver is an incredible organ that works tirelessly to protect you from the constant barrage of toxins you encounter daily. However, much like a machine, it needs maintenance. By recognising the signs of liver stress and taking steps to support its detox functions—through diet, hydration, exercise, and possibly supplements—you can help ensure that your liver remains healthy and able to do its vital work for years to come.

Summary: Introduction to Liver Health and Detoxification

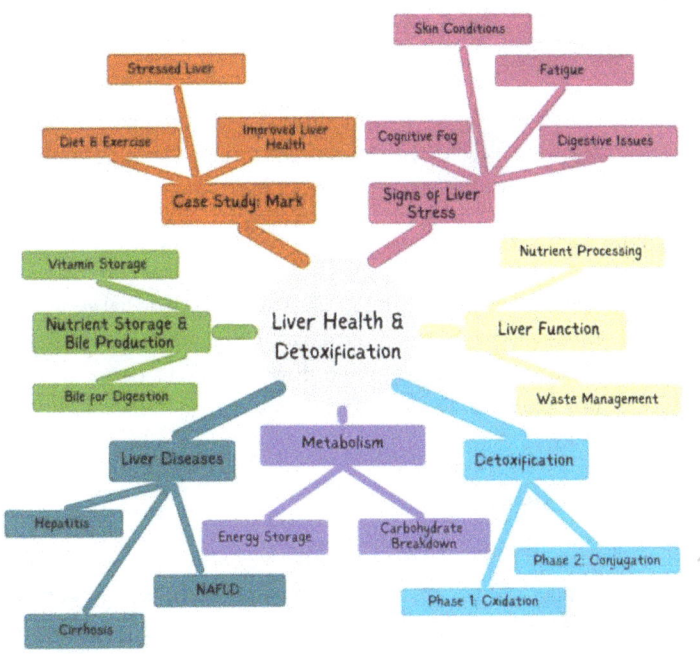

Chapter 2
The Science Behind Liver Detox

In this chapter, we will dive deeper into **how liver detoxification works**, why it is essential, and the science behind it. The liver plays a vital role in neutralising harmful substances and ensuring your body runs smoothly. Understanding how the liver handles toxins and what happens when it is overwhelmed can help you make informed decisions about supporting liver health.

Toxins and Liver Health

Imagine your liver as a diligent factory worker, sorting through the raw materials (nutrients) that enter your body and processing the waste (toxins). These toxins come from various sources:

1. **Environmental Toxins**:

    These include pollutants in the air, pesticides, and chemicals found in cleaning products or even skincare. You can think of them as the "smog" that your liver has to filter out.

2. **Dietary Toxins**:

    These toxins arise from processed foods, artificial additives, excess sugar, and unhealthy fats. Over time, a diet high in these substances can weigh down the liver's detox system, just like running a machine on low-quality fuel can cause it to break down.

3. **Internal Toxins**:

    Beyond external toxins, your body produces waste products during normal metabolism. For instance, when proteins break down, they create **ammonia**, which is highly toxic. It is your liver's job to convert ammonia into **urea**, which can then be safely excreted in urine. If your liver isn't functioning well, these internal toxins can build up, contributing to fatigue, headaches, and other symptoms.

In essence, the liver is your body's waste treatment plant. The more toxins you're exposed to—whether from food, your environment, or metabolic processes—the harder the liver has to work to keep your system clean.

The Role of Inflammation

When toxins accumulate faster than the liver can process them, **inflammation** begins to set in. Think of inflammation as your body's internal alarm system—when something harmful is detected, your immune system reacts by releasing chemicals that cause swelling and redness in affected areas. While short-term inflammation helps the body heal, chronic inflammation can be damaging, especially to the liver.

- **Chronic Liver Inflammation:**

    Chronic inflammation occurs when the liver is consistently exposed to toxins and cannot clear them quickly enough. The immune system remains on high alert, continuously sending out inflammatory signals. Over time, this can lead to scarring of the liver tissue, known as **fibrosis**, and in severe cases, **cirrhosis**.

- **Systemic Inflammation:**

    Inflammation in the liver does not stay confined to that organ. It often spreads throughout the body, leading to problems like **metabolic syndrome, type 2 diabetes**, and even **heart disease.** It is as if a fire started in one room of a house but quickly spread to other rooms. Addressing liver inflammation early on can prevent these broader health issues.

To reduce liver inflammation, it is crucial to eliminate or limit your exposure to toxins. This could mean choosing organic foods, avoiding processed snacks, and staying hydrated to help your liver flush out toxins more effectively.

How Liver Detox Works

Now that we know what the liver is up against, let us break down how liver detoxification works. It is essential to understand that "detox" does not mean you need to follow a strict juice cleanse or drink special teas. In reality, your liver is detoxifying all the time; it just needs the right tools and support to function at its best.

As we touched on in **Chapter 1**, liver detox occurs in **two phases**:

- **Phase 1: Breaking Down Toxins**

    During Phase 1, the liver's enzymes, especially the **cytochrome P450 enzymes**, transform toxins into more water-soluble molecules. However, these new molecules are often even more reactive and potentially harmful in their intermediate state—like converting a mild irritant into something more dangerous before it can be neutralised. To manage this process, the liver relies on **antioxidants** (such as **glutathione**) to prevent damage.

- **Phase 2: Making Toxins Safe**

    In Phase 2, these reactive intermediates are neutralised. The liver attaches molecules like **glutathione**, **sulfate**, or **glycine** to them, rendering the toxins harmless. Once neutralised, these toxins can be safely excreted through urine or bile. Think of this step as wrapping toxic waste in a protective package, ensuring it can be thrown away without causing harm.

For this detox process to work smoothly, the liver needs a constant supply of specific nutrients, including:

- **Antioxidants** like vitamins **C** and **E**
- **B vitamins** to support enzymatic activity
- **Amino acids** (from protein) to form molecules like glutathione

Without these nutrients, the liver struggles to keep up with the detox load, leaving harmful toxins circulating in the body.

Lifestyle Factors that Impact Liver Detox

Your daily habits play a huge role in how well your liver can perform its detox duties. Several lifestyle factors can either help or hinder this process:

1. **Diet:**

    A diet rich in fresh vegetables, fruits, lean proteins, and whole grains provides the essential nutrients your liver needs. Foods like **broccoli, garlic, beets,** and **leafy greens** contain compounds that actively support the liver's detox functions.

    Conversely, a diet high in processed foods, sugars, and unhealthy fats places a burden on the liver, as these substances are harder to break down and often create more harmful by-products. It is like giving your liver low-quality fuel that creates more residue, causing the engine to work harder.

2. **Hydration:**

    Drinking enough water is essential for the liver to flush out toxins efficiently. Imagine trying to wash dishes without enough water—you won't be able to clean them thoroughly. Staying well-hydrated ensures that toxins are diluted and easily excreted via urine.

3. **Alcohol and Smoking**:

    Both alcohol and tobacco products introduce a significant toxin load to the liver. **Alcohol,** in particular, puts immense pressure on the liver's detox pathways. Even moderate drinking can interfere with the liver's ability to break down other toxins. Over time, excessive alcohol use can lead to **alcoholic liver disease**, where liver cells become inflamed and die.

4. **Stress**:

    High stress levels can lead to hormone imbalances, causing the liver to work harder to break down excess stress hormones like **cortisol**. Chronic stress may also lead to unhealthy coping mechanisms, such as overeating or drinking alcohol, which further burden the liver.

How to Support Liver Detox

Supporting liver detox does not have to be complicated. There are several practical steps you can take to give your liver the nutrients and rest it needs:

1. **Eat Liver-Supportive Foods**:

    Incorporating more detox-friendly foods into your diet can provide the liver with the nutrients it needs. **Cruciferous vegetables** like broccoli and kale contain sulfur compounds that enhance the liver's ability to detoxify harmful chemicals. **Garlic** is also a great addition to your meals, as it is rich in **selenium** and **allicin,** which boost the liver's detox function.

2. **Stay Hydrated**:

    Drinking at least 8 glasses of water a day will help your liver flush out toxins and support the kidneys in removing waste products. Herbal teas, such as **dandelion root tea**, are also beneficial because they promote bile production and help the liver digest fats more effectively.

3. **Exercise:**

   Regular physical activity can help improve liver function. Exercise increases blood circulation, allowing the liver to filter more blood and eliminate toxins. It also reduces **visceral fat**, which is closely linked to liver diseases like NAFLD.

4. **Limit Alcohol and Smoking:**

   Reducing or eliminating alcohol and cigarettes from your routine will immediately reduce the toxic load on your liver. Your liver will thank you for the break from processing these harmful substances!

5. **Manage Stress:**

   Incorporating stress management techniques such as **meditation, yoga**, or **deep breathing exercises** can help reduce the burden on your liver. Less stress means fewer stress hormones for the liver to metabolise.

Case History: Managing Inflammation with Liver Detox

Background:

Anna, a 35-year-old woman, began experiencing chronic fatigue, joint pain, and digestive discomfort. After ruling out autoimmune conditions, her doctor suspected that long-term inflammation caused by poor liver detox could be contributing to her symptoms. A blood test revealed elevated **C-reactive protein (CRP)**, a marker of inflammation, as well as mild liver inflammation.

The Detox Plan:

Anna started a liver detox program focused on reducing inflammation:

1. **Diet**: She eliminated processed foods and incorporated more anti-inflammatory foods like leafy greens, berries, and fish high in **omega-3 fatty acids**.

2. **Supplements**: She added **glutathione** and **turmeric** (which contains the anti-inflammatory compound curcumin) to her daily routine.

3. **Lifestyle Changes**: She made an effort to stay hydrated and engage in moderate exercise 5 times a week.

Results:

Within three months, Anna's CRP levels dropped significantly, and she reported improved energy and less digestive discomfort. Her liver inflammation markers also returned to normal, showing that the detox program had helped restore balance.

Conclusion

Your liver is your body's natural detox powerhouse, but it needs support to function optimally, especially in your liver is your body's natural detox powerhouse, but it needs support to function optimally, especially in today's world, where we are exposed to more environmental toxins than ever before. Understanding how the liver processes these toxins, what causes inflammation, and how to incorporate lifestyle changes can help you maintain a healthy, efficient liver.

Just as you wouldn't let trash pile up in your house, you shouldn't let toxins accumulate in your body. By managing your diet, reducing stress, and staying hydrated, you can keep your liver functioning at its best, supporting your overall health and well-being.

Liver Revival

Summary: The Science Behind Liver Detox

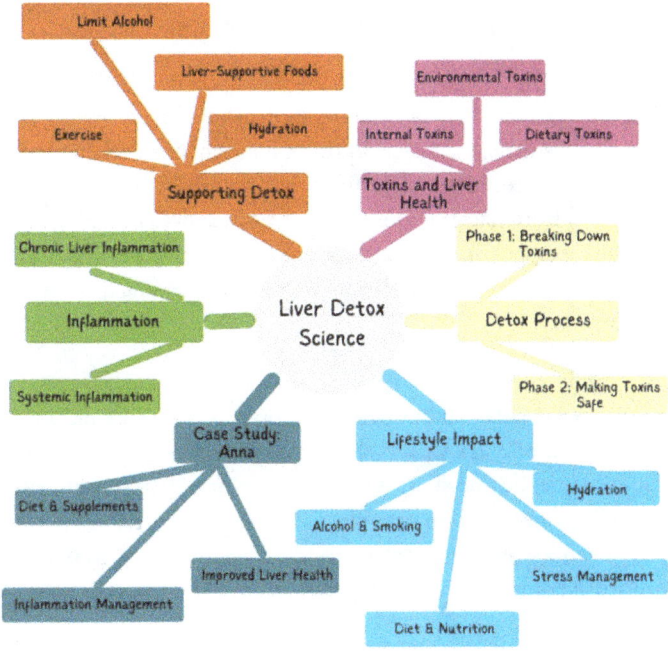

Chapter 3
Pharmacological Approaches to Liver Detox

The liver is an incredibly resilient organ, capable of regenerating itself even after sustaining damage. However, there are times when modern medicine is needed to give it extra support, especially when detoxifying from harmful substances or treating liver-related diseases. In these cases, pharmacological approaches can play a crucial role in helping the liver process and eliminate toxins, prevent damage, and promote recovery.

In this chapter, we'll explore how specific medications and treatments can aid the liver's detoxification process. These include **N-acetylcysteine (NAC)**, **S-adenosylmethionine (SAMe)**, **ursodeoxycholic acid (UDCA)**, **Tauroursodeoxycholic acid (TUDCA)**, and chelation therapies for heavy metal detox. When used in conjunction with lifestyle changes, these treatments can significantly improve liver function and help people recover from toxin overload.

Prescription Medications for Liver Health

Pharmaceutical interventions can directly support liver detox by enhancing its capacity to neutralise toxins, regenerate cells, or improve bile flow. Below are some of the most common medications used to protect and detoxify the liver:

- **N-acetylcysteine (NAC):**

    NAC is a powerful antioxidant that increases levels of **glutathione**, the liver's primary defence against toxins. Glutathione acts like a sponge, soaking up free radicals and harmful substances before they can damage liver cells. NAC is commonly used in hospitals to treat **acetaminophen (paracetamol) overdoses**, a leading cause of acute liver failure. By replenishing glutathione, NAC helps the liver neutralise toxins and recover more quickly from injury.

Analogy: Imagine your liver as a water filter that gets clogged over time. NAC works like a cleaning agent, removing the blockages and allowing the filter (your liver) to process water (toxins) more efficiently again.

- **S-adenosylmethionine (SAMe)**:

    SAMe is a naturally occurring compound in the body that helps with detoxification, inflammation control, and cell regeneration. It is especially useful in treating **fatty liver disease** and **cirrhosis**, where liver cells are damaged and inflamed. SAMe supports the liver by aiding in **methylation**, a critical process for detoxification, and by reducing oxidative stress. It is also used as an antidepressant, which can be helpful in cases where liver damage is linked to stress or depression.

- **Ursodeoxycholic Acid (UDCA)**:

    UDCA is a bile acid that helps improve bile flow, which is crucial for detoxification. When bile flow is impaired (as in conditions like **primary biliary cholangitis** or **gallstones**), toxins can accumulate in the liver. UDCA helps reduce liver inflammation, protect bile ducts, and promote better digestion and toxin elimination. It is like unclogging a drain—by allowing bile to flow freely, UDCA prevents a backup of toxins that could further damage the liver.

TUDCA: A Bile Acid for Liver Detox

Tauroursodeoxycholic acid (TUDCA) is another bile acid with significant benefits for liver health. It has been used for centuries in traditional Chinese medicine. It is now recognised for its role in treating **cholestasis** (impaired bile flow) and other liver conditions. TUDCA protects liver cells from bile acid-induced damage and promotes healthier bile flow, reducing the buildup of harmful substances in the liver.

- **How TUDCA Works:**

    TUDCA helps the liver by improving bile flow and preventing the accumulation of toxic bile acids that can damage liver cells. It also has **anti-apoptotic** properties, meaning it can prevent liver cell death, which is critical in conditions like **non-alcoholic fatty liver disease (NAFLD)** and **alcoholic liver disease**.

- **Benefits of TUDCA:**

    a. **Improves Bile Flow**: TUDCA helps ensure that bile flows freely, preventing toxins from being trapped in the liver.

    b. **Reduces Inflammation**: TUDCA has anti-inflammatory properties that help reduce liver damage caused by chronic inflammation.

    c. **Prevents Liver Cell Death**: TUDCA protects liver cells from damage, preserving liver function in patients with bile flow issues or toxin overload.

- **Case History: TUDCA for Cholestasis**

    Background:

    Sarah, a 40-year-old woman diagnosed with **primary biliary cholangitis (PBC)**, was experiencing symptoms such as fatigue, itching, and jaundice due to impaired bile flow. Her initial treatment with UDCA showed limited improvement, so her doctor added **TUDCA** to her regimen.

Treatment Plan:

Sarah was prescribed 500 mg of TUDCA daily alongside UDCA to help improve bile flow and reduce liver inflammation.

Results:

After three months, Sarah's symptoms improved significantly, with reduced itching and better energy levels. Follow-up blood tests showed a decrease in liver enzymes, indicating improved liver function.

Medications for Heavy Metal Detox

Heavy metals like **mercury, lead,** and **cadmium** are particularly toxic to the liver because they accumulate over time and are difficult for the body to eliminate. This is where **chelating agents** come into play. These medications bind to metals in the bloodstream and help the body excrete them.

- **Chelation Therapy with EDTA:**

    Ethylenediaminetetraacetic acid (EDTA) is a common chelating agent used to treat **lead poisoning** and other heavy metal exposures. It binds to metals, allowing them to be excreted through urine. Chelation therapy is typically administered under medical supervision because it can also remove essential minerals, so patients often need **mineral supplements** to restore balance.

Analogy: Heavy metals in your body are like gum stuck in a machine's gears. Chelation therapy acts like a solvent that dissolves the gum, allowing the machine (your liver) to function smoothly again.

- **DMSA and DMPS:**

    DMSA (Dimercaptosuccinic acid) and **DMPS (Dimercaptopropane sulfonate)** are other chelating agents used to detoxify the body from mercury and other metals. These compounds bind to heavy metals, making them easier for the kidneys to excrete. DMSA is typically administered orally, while DMPS may be given intravenously for more rapid detoxification.

- **IV Glutathione for Heavy Metal Detox:**

    In addition to chelation agents, **glutathione** can be administered intravenously to help the liver cope with the oxidative stress caused by heavy metals. IV glutathione allows for quick delivery of this powerful antioxidant, helping neutralise the free radicals produced during detoxification.

Risks and Side Effects

While pharmacological approaches to liver detox are highly effective, they can also have side effects if not carefully managed:

- **Nutrient Depletion:**

    Chelation therapy can remove not only harmful metals but also essential minerals like calcium, zinc, and magnesium. Patients undergoing chelation therapy should take mineral supplements to prevent deficiencies that could impair liver function or lead to other health issues, such as muscle cramps, fatigue, or immune suppression.

Analogy: It is like using a powerful cleaning agent that not only removes stains but also strips away the paint. Without the right precautions, chelation therapy can deplete the body of vital nutrients.

- **Over-reliance on Pharmaceuticals:**

    Pharmaceuticals can be an important part of liver detox, especially in acute cases like heavy metal poisoning or alcohol-related liver damage. However, relying solely on medication without addressing lifestyle factors—such as poor diet, lack of exercise, and ongoing exposure to toxins—can limit the effectiveness of these treatments.

Supporting Liver Health with Lifestyle Changes

Medications can be incredibly effective at supporting liver detox, but they work best when combined with lifestyle changes. Here are some simple but powerful steps you can take to support your liver while undergoing pharmacological treatment:

1. **Eat a Liver-Supporting Diet:**

    A diet rich in leafy greens, cruciferous vegetables (like broccoli and Brussels sprouts), and healthy fats (like olive oil and avocados) provides the liver with the nutrients it needs to detoxify effectively. Garlic and onions are beneficial, as they contain sulfur compounds that boost liver detox enzymes.

2. **Stay Hydrated:**

    Drinking plenty of water helps your body flush out toxins more effectively. Staying hydrated supports both the kidneys and liver in removing waste products from the body. Aim for at least eight glasses of water a day.

3. **Exercise Regularly:**

    Regular exercise increases blood flow, allowing the liver to filter more blood and remove toxins. Exercise also helps reduce excess fat in the liver, which is particularly important for individuals with **non-alcoholic fatty liver disease (NAFLD)**.

4. **Limit Alcohol and Processed Foods:**

    Alcohol places a heavy burden on the liver. Hence, reducing or eliminating it from your diet is essential during a liver detox. Processed foods, particularly those high in sugar and trans fats, can also overload the liver, slowing down the detox process.

Case History: Alcohol-Induced Liver Damage and Pharmacological Support

Case History: Alcohol-Induced Liver Damage and Pharmacological Support

Background:

John, a 52-year-old man, had been drinking regularly for over two decades. Over time, he noticed increasing fatigue, digestive issues, and frequent headaches. After experiencing chronic symptoms, a routine blood test revealed elevated liver enzyme levels (**ALT** and **AST**), indicating significant stress on his liver, primarily from long-term alcohol consumption. His doctor explained that continued alcohol use could lead to more severe conditions, such as **cirrhosis**.

Treatment Plan:

John's doctor recommended a liver detox program that combined pharmaceutical treatments and lifestyle changes. To support his liver's recovery, he was prescribed **N-acetylcysteine (NAC)** to increase **glutathione** production and help his liver neutralise the toxins produced by years of alcohol use. Alongside this, he was prescribed **S-adenosylmethionine (SAMe)** to support liver regeneration and reduce inflammation.

Since alcohol impairs bile flow, leading to further accumulation of toxins, John's doctor also added **ursodeoxycholic acid (UDCA)** to help improve bile flow and protect the liver from damage caused by bile acid buildup. UDCA would also help prevent further liver cell damage by enhancing the natural bile flow pathways and reducing the risk of bile buildup.

Lifestyle Changes:

In addition to his medication regimen, John made significant lifestyle changes. He completely eliminated alcohol and switched to a liver-friendly diet rich in leafy greens, lean proteins, and whole grains. He incorporated liver-supportive foods like garlic, spinach, and beets, known for their high antioxidant content. He also committed to walking daily and drinking plenty of water to stay hydrated.

Results:

After six months, John's liver enzyme levels dropped to normal, and his overall energy levels improved. His doctor noted a reduction in liver inflammation and emphasised that the combination of **NAC**, **SAMe**, and **UDCA**, along with John's lifestyle changes, had significantly improved his liver function. The successful reduction in enzyme levels indicated that the liver had begun to heal from years of damage.

Conclusion

Pharmacological approaches offer valuable support for liver detox, especially in cases of chronic liver disease, heavy metal toxicity, or prolonged toxin exposure from alcohol and medications. Medications like **N-acetylcysteine (NAC)**, **S-adenosylmethionine (SAMe)**, **TUDCA**, and **chelating agents** help the liver recover and function more efficiently by replenishing essential detoxifying substances, improving bile flow, and protecting liver cells from damage.

However, medications are most effective when combined with lifestyle changes. A diet rich in nutrients, regular exercise, adequate hydration, and avoiding alcohol and processed foods are crucial for long-term liver health. Much like maintaining a car with regular oil changes and clean fuel, these lifestyle adjustments ensure the liver continues running smoothly and efficiently.

By supporting your liver with the proper medications and healthy habits, you can significantly improve your body's ability to detoxify harmful substances, prevent liver damage, and promote overall well-being.

Summary: Pharmacological Approaches to Liver Detox

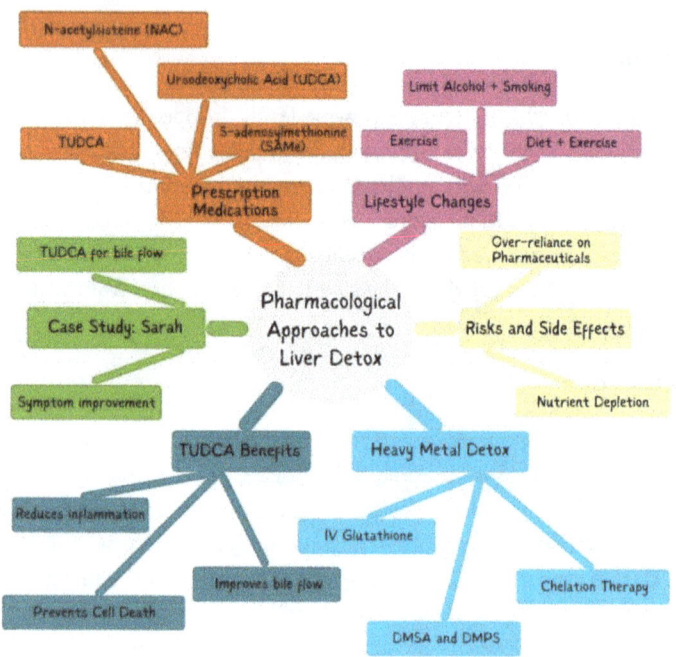

Chapter 4
Micronutrients for Liver Health

Micronutrients, including vitamins, minerals, and antioxidants, are essential for liver health. They play a crucial role in the liver's ability to detoxify harmful substances, regenerate healthy cells, and perform its wide range of metabolic functions.

In this chapter, we'll explore the key micronutrients that support liver health, how they work, and why you need to make sure you're getting enough of them through your diet or supplementation.

The Role of Micronutrients in Liver Detoxification

The liver's ability to detoxify harmful substances largely depends on a complex network of enzymes and biochemical reactions, all of which require specific vitamins and minerals to function optimally. These micronutrients are like the tools in a mechanic's toolbox—without them, the liver can't effectively process toxins.

1. **Vitamins**:

    Vitamins like **A, D, E, K**, and **B vitamins** are crucial for liver health. They help the liver process fats, convert toxins into water-soluble compounds, and protect liver cells from oxidative damage.

2. **Minerals**:

    Minerals like **zinc, selenium,** and **magnesium** serve as cofactors for many liver enzymes. Without these minerals, key detoxification processes, such as neutralising free radicals, cannot take place effectively.

3. **Antioxidants:**

> **Glutathione** is the liver's most powerful antioxidant, protecting cells from the oxidative stress caused by free radicals. Other antioxidants, like **vitamin C** and **vitamin E**, help replenish glutathione and protect liver cells from damage.

Key Micronutrients for Liver Health

Glutathione: The Master Antioxidant

- **Function:**

    > Glutathione is a tripeptide made up of three amino acids: **glutamine, glycine,** and **cysteine**. It plays a critical role in neutralising free radicals, detoxifying harmful substances, and supporting the liver's Phase 2 detoxification process. Essentially, glutathione binds to toxins and makes them water-soluble, so they can be easily excreted from the body through bile or urine.

Analogy: Think of glutathione as the liver's "sponge," soaking up harmful toxins before they can damage cells. When glutathione levels are depleted, the liver struggles to process toxins, much like a dry sponge that can't absorb any more water.

- **Food Sources:**

    > Foods rich in **sulfur-containing amino acids** (such as garlic, onions, and cruciferous vegetables) help boost glutathione production. Other helpful foods include spinach, avocados, and asparagus.

- **Supplementation:**

    Glutathione can be taken as a supplement, but it is often more effective to supplement with **N-acetylcysteine (NAC)**, which helps the body produce more glutathione naturally.

B Vitamins: Supporting Detox Enzymes

- **Function:**

    The **B vitamin complex**, particularly **B6, B12**, and **folate**, is critical for the liver's methylation process, which helps detoxify harmful substances. B vitamins are also involved in the production of glutathione and support energy production in the liver. Without adequate B vitamins, the liver's detox pathways (Phase 1 and Phase 2) become sluggish, leading to toxin buildup.

Analogy: Imagine B vitamins as the fuel that powers the liver's detoxification engines. Without enough fuel, the engines (detox pathways) slow down, allowing toxins to accumulate in the body.

- **Food Sources:**

    You can find B vitamins in a wide range of foods, including leafy greens (folate), meat, eggs, and dairy (B12), and legumes (B6).

- **Supplementation:**

    People with liver disease or those who don't eat enough B-vitamin-rich foods may benefit from B-complex supplements to ensure they're getting enough of these essential nutrients.

Liver Revival

Selenium: The Liver's Detox Cofactor

- **Function:**

    Selenium is an essential trace mineral that helps activate **glutathione peroxidase**. This enzyme plays a crucial role in detoxifying harmful substances and protecting liver cells from oxidative damage. Selenium also aids in the regeneration of glutathione, ensuring that the liver has enough antioxidant power to neutralise toxins.

Analogy: Think of selenium as the key that turns on your liver's detoxification machinery. Without it, detox enzymes can't function effectively, leaving toxins to build up in your system.

- **Food Sources:**

    One of the richest sources of selenium is **Brazil nuts**—just one or two per day can provide your recommended daily intake. Other sources include fish, eggs, and sunflower seeds.

- **Supplementation:**

    People who are selenium deficient may benefit from selenium supplements, but it is important not to exceed recommended doses, as too much selenium can be harmful.

Zinc: Essential for Liver Enzymes

- **Function:**
Zinc is another vital mineral that supports liver health by aiding in the production of enzymes that detoxify alcohol and other toxins. Zinc is also involved in protecting the liver from inflammation and oxidative damage.

Analogy: Think of zinc as the wrench that tightens the liver's detoxification systems. Without it, the detox machinery becomes loose and ineffective.

- **Food Sources:**

    Zinc-rich foods include shellfish (especially oysters), red meat, seeds, and legumes.

- **Supplementation:**

    Zinc supplements can be beneficial, especially for people with liver disease or those who consume a diet low in zinc-rich foods. However, like selenium, zinc should be taken in appropriate amounts, as too much zinc can interfere with the absorption of other important minerals.

Food Sources vs. Supplements

While it is always ideal to get your vitamins and minerals from whole foods, there are times when supplementation is necessary. People with liver conditions, nutrient deficiencies, or restrictive diets may need supplements to ensure they're getting enough micronutrients to support liver function.

1. **Getting Nutrients from Food:**

    The liver thrives on a diet rich in fruits, vegetables, lean proteins, and healthy fats. Whole foods not only provide essential vitamins and minerals, but they also contain fibre and other compounds that support digestion and overall liver health. For example, **cruciferous vegetables** like broccoli and Brussels sprouts contain compounds called **glucosinolates**, which enhance the liver's ability to detoxify harmful substances.

2. **Supplementation:**

    In cases where people have liver disease or are unable to absorb enough nutrients from food, supplements can help fill in the gaps. Supplements like **glutathione**, **NAC**, **selenium**, and **B vitamins** are commonly recommended to support liver health. However, it is important to consult a healthcare provider before starting any new supplement regimen, as too much of certain nutrients can be harmful.

Micronutrient Deficiencies and Liver Disease

Micronutrient deficiencies are common in people with liver disease. The liver plays a key role in absorbing and storing vitamins and minerals, but when it is damaged, its ability to process these nutrients is compromised. Here are some common deficiencies associated with liver disease:

- **Vitamin D Deficiency:**

    People with liver disease are often deficient in **vitamin D**, which is important for bone health and immune function. Supplementing with vitamin D can help improve liver function and reduce inflammation.

- **Zinc Deficiency:**

    Zinc deficiency is common in people with chronic liver disease and can lead to further liver damage. Supplementing with zinc can help reduce inflammation and support the liver's detox processes.

- **Selenium Deficiency:**

    Selenium deficiency is linked to increased oxidative stress in the liver, which can worsen liver conditions like **NAFLD** and **cirrhosis**. Supplementing with selenium can help protect liver cells and support detoxification.

Case History: Micronutrient Deficiency and Liver Health

Background:

Sarah, a 45-year-old woman, had been diagnosed with **non-alcoholic fatty liver disease (NAFLD)** after years of consuming a diet high in processed foods and sugar. She felt constantly fatigued and struggled with frequent brain fog, bloating, and weight gain. Her blood tests revealed that she had low levels of **vitamin D, zinc,** and **selenium.**

The Plan:

Sarah's doctor recommended a diet overhaul to support liver detox and address her nutrient deficiencies. She was advised to incorporate more leafy greens, cruciferous vegetables, and lean proteins into her meals. Additionally, she was prescribed supplements for **vitamin D, zinc,** and **selenium**, along with **N-acetylcysteine (NAC)** to boost glutathione levels.

Results:

Within three months, Sarah's energy levels improved, and her brain fog diminished. Follow-up blood tests showed that her liver enzymes had normalised, and her micronutrient levels were back in the healthy range. By addressing her nutrient deficiencies and supporting her liver's detox pathways, Sarah was able to reverse the early stages of NAFLD and improve her overall health.

Conclusion

Micronutrients play a crucial role in supporting liver detoxification and overall liver health. Ensuring that your diet is rich in vitamins, minerals, and antioxidants is essential for maintaining liver function, especially in the face of modern-day toxin exposure. While food is the best source of these nutrients, supplements may be necessary for people with liver disease or nutrient deficiencies. By supporting your liver with the right nutrients, you give it the tools it needs to detoxify efficiently and regenerate healthy cells.

Micronutrient deficiencies, especially in key nutrients like glutathione, B vitamins, selenium, and zinc, can impair the liver's ability to detoxify harmful substances, leading to fatigue, inflammation, and liver damage. However, by incorporating liver-supportive foods and supplements, you can help your liver function at its best, preventing long-term damage and improving overall health.

Chapter Summary:

This chapter explored the essential micronutrients that support liver health, focusing on their roles in detoxification, regeneration, and protection from oxidative stress. We covered the importance of **glutathione**, **B vitamins**, **selenium**, and **zinc**, and how deficiencies in these nutrients can negatively impact liver function. We also discussed how you can obtain these nutrients from food and when supplementation might be necessary. The case history illustrated how addressing micronutrient deficiencies can help reverse liver damage, highlighting the critical role that nutrition plays in liver detox.

Summary: Micronutrients for Liver Health

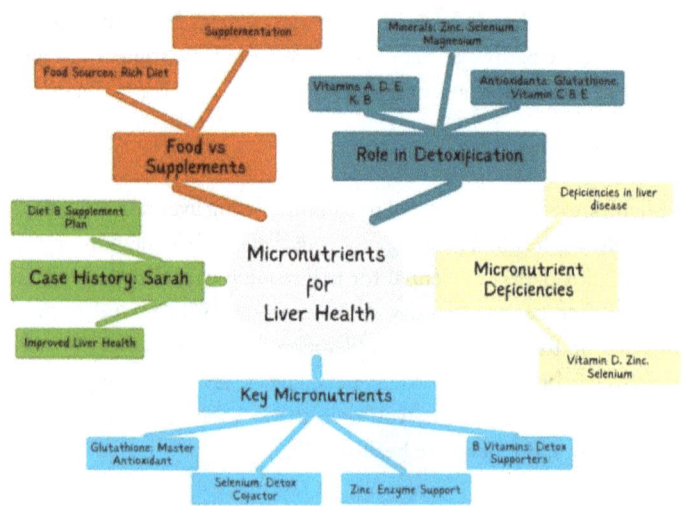

Chapter 5
Herbal and Botanical Support for Liver Detox

Throughout history, herbal remedies have been used to support liver health and detoxification. Many of these herbs are still widely used today, and modern science has validated their effectiveness through research and clinical studies. In this chapter, we'll explore the most well-known herbs that support liver detox, how they work, and how you can incorporate them into your daily routine.

We'll also discuss the difference between traditional uses of these herbs and the modern scientific understanding, blending ancient wisdom with today's evidence-based practices.

Popul   ar Herbs for Liver Detox

Herbs are nature's medicine, and certain herbs have long been known to have hepatoprotective (liver-protecting) properties. These herbs work in various ways, from boosting bile production to supporting the liver's antioxidant defences. Let us take a closer look at some of the most widely used herbs for liver health.

Milk Thistle (Silybum marianum)

- **Function:**

    Milk thistle is one of the most extensively studied herbs for liver health. Its active ingredient, **silymarin**, has been shown to have antioxidant, anti-inflammatory, and antifibrotic (anti-scarring) properties. Silymarin helps protect liver cells by stabilising their cell membranes and promoting protein synthesis, which aids in liver regeneration. Milk thistle is often used to treat conditions such as **fatty liver disease**, **cirrhosis**, and **hepatitis**.

Analogy: Imagine the liver as a sponge. Over time, toxins can damage the sponge, making it less effective. Milk thistle acts like a protective coating, shielding the sponge from damage while helping it repair itself.

- **Scientific Evidence:**

    Several studies have demonstrated the hepatoprotective effects of milk thistle. A review of clinical trials found that silymarin reduced liver enzyme levels in patients with chronic liver disease and improved overall liver function. Another study showed that silymarin could reduce liver damage caused by alcohol, making it a popular herb for those recovering from alcohol-related liver issues.

- **How to Use:**

    Milk thistle is available as a supplement in capsule or tincture form. It can also be consumed as a tea, although the concentration of silymarin in tea may be lower than in standardised supplements. The typical dose is 200–400 mg of silymarin per day, but it is important to consult a healthcare provider before starting any new supplement.

Turmeric (Curcuma longa)

- **Function:**

    Turmeric, particularly its active compound **curcumin**, has powerful anti-inflammatory and antioxidant properties. It supports liver detoxification by boosting the production of bile, which helps the liver break down and remove toxins. Curcumin also helps reduce liver inflammation, making it useful for managing conditions like **non-alcoholic fatty liver disease (NAFLD)** and liver inflammation due to toxin overload.

Analogy: Think of turmeric as a firefighter for the liver—it helps extinguish the flames of inflammation and protects liver cells from further damage.

- **Scientific Evidence:**

    Several studies have shown that curcumin can reduce inflammation and oxidative stress in the liver. A 2019 clinical trial found that patients with NAFLD who took curcumin supplements experienced significant improvements in liver enzyme levels and reductions in liver fat. Another study demonstrated curcumin's ability to inhibit inflammatory pathways, particularly **NF-kB**, a molecule that plays a key role in liver inflammation.

- **How to Use:**

    Turmeric can be consumed as a spice in food or taken as a supplement. For liver health, curcumin supplements are often preferred, as they provide a higher concentration of the active compound. Turmeric supplements typically contain **piperine** (from black pepper) to enhance curcumin absorption. The standard dose for curcumin is 500–1,000 mg per day.

Dandelion Root (Taraxacum officinale)

- **Function:**

    Dandelion root has been used for centuries to promote liver detoxification and support bile production. It acts as a mild diuretic, helping the body eliminate excess fluids and toxins. By stimulating bile production, dandelion root enhances fat digestion and helps the liver excrete fat-soluble toxins. It is often used as a gentle detox herb, especially for those with sluggish digestion or liver congestion.

Analogy: Think of dandelion root as a "spring cleaning" herb for the liver—it helps sweep out toxins and stimulates the liver to work more efficiently.

- **Scientific Evidence:**

    While scientific research on dandelion root is limited compared to other herbs, some studies suggest that it has hepatoprotective effects. One animal study found that dandelion root extract reduced oxidative stress and inflammation in the liver, potentially protecting against liver injury. Traditional uses of dandelion root as a liver tonic are supported by its ability to stimulate bile flow.

- **How to Use:**

    Dandelion root can be consumed as a tea, tincture, or capsule. Many people enjoy dandelion tea as part of a daily detox regimen. A typical dose for dandelion root capsules is 500–1,000 mg per day.

Schisandra (Schisandra chinensis)

- **Function:**

    Schisandra is an adaptogenic herb used in **Traditional Chinese Medicine (TCM)** to support liver function and protect against liver damage. It is known for its ability to increase the production of liver detox enzymes and enhance the liver's antioxidant defences. Schisandra also helps regulate liver function, making it particularly useful for those experiencing liver stress from environmental toxins or overwork.

Analogy: Schisandra acts like a stress manager for the liver, helping it cope with overloads of toxins and improving its ability to handle stress.

- **Scientific Evidence:**

    Studies have shown that schisandra extract can increase the activity of **glutathione** and other antioxidant enzymes in the liver. This helps reduce oxidative stress and inflammation, protecting liver cells from damage. Schisandra has also been studied for its ability to improve liver enzyme levels and promote the regeneration of damaged liver tissue.

- **How to Use:**

    Schisandra is commonly available in capsule, tincture, or powdered form. It can be added to smoothies, teas, or taken as a supplement. The standard dose is 500–1,500 mg per day, depending on the form used.

Artichoke Leaf (Cynara scolymus)

- **Function:**

Artichoke leaf is known for its ability to stimulate bile production and support liver detoxification. It contains **cynarin**, a compound that increases bile flow, aiding in digestion and the excretion of fat-soluble toxins. Artichoke leaf is particularly useful for improving digestion and reducing symptoms of bloating and indigestion associated with poor liver function.

Analogy: Artichoke leaf acts like a digestive aid for the liver, helping it process fats more efficiently and ensuring that toxins are flushed out effectively.

- **Scientific Evidence:**

    A 2018 study found that artichoke extract improved liver enzyme levels in patients with NAFLD and reduced fat accumulation in the liver. Another study showed that artichoke leaf extract could reduce cholesterol levels and improve bile secretion, supporting the liver's ability to detoxify the body.

- **How to Use:**

    Artichoke leaf is typically taken as a supplement in capsule or tincture form. The usual dose is 300–500 mg of artichoke extract per day.

Liver Revival

Traditional Use vs. Modern Science

Many of the herbs used for liver detox have been employed for centuries in traditional medicine systems such as Ayurveda and Traditional Chinese Medicine (TCM). While modern science has validated the effectiveness of many of these herbs, it is interesting to see how traditional wisdom aligns with contemporary research.

- **Traditional Use:**

    In TCM, herbs like **schisandra** and **milk thistle** have long been used to support liver health, promote longevity, and protect against disease. In Ayurveda, detoxifying herbs like **turmeric** and **dandelion root** are often used as part of a cleansing program known as **Panchakarma**, which aims to remove toxins (ama) from the body and restore balance.

- **Modern Science:**

    Today, we understand more about the specific biochemical pathways these herbs support. For example, we now know that turmeric's anti-inflammatory properties stem from its ability to inhibit the **NF-kB** pathway, and that milk thistle's silymarin protects liver cells from oxidative damage. Modern extraction techniques also allow us to concentrate the active compounds in these herbs, making them more potent and effective.

Case History: Herbal Detox Success Story

Background:

Tom, a 50-year-old man, had been struggling with mild **non-alcoholic fatty liver disease (NAFLD)** for several years. He frequently experienced bloating, fatigue, and occasional discomfort after eating. His blood tests showed elevated liver enzymes, indicating liver stress. Tom wasn't ready to rely on prescription medications and wanted to explore natural alternatives to support his liver health.

The Plan:

Tom's healthcare provider recommended a comprehensive liver detox program that included a combination of herbal supplements. He started taking **milk thistle** to promote liver cell regeneration and reduce liver enzyme levels, **turmeric** for its anti-inflammatory effects, and **dandelion root** to support bile production and digestion. In addition, Tom incorporated **artichoke leaf extract** into his routine to enhance bile flow and improve fat digestion.

Results:

After three months of using these herbal supplements and making minor dietary adjustments, Tom's liver enzyme levels had significantly improved, dropping back into the normal range. He reported feeling more energised, less bloated, and able to digest meals more comfortably. His healthcare provider suggested that Tom continue using these herbs to maintain liver health and prevent further fat accumulation in the liver.

Incorporating Herbs into Your Liver Detox Routine

Incorporating liver-supportive herbs into your daily routine can be an easy and effective way to support your body's natural detoxification processes. Here are some simple ways to add these herbs to your diet:

1. **Herbal Teas:**

    Many liver-supporting herbs, like **dandelion root** and **turmeric**, can be consumed as teas. Drinking a cup of **dandelion root tea** or **milk thistle tea** daily is a simple and effective way to support liver detox.

2. **Capsules and Supplements:**

    If you prefer not to drink teas or want a more concentrated dose, most liver-supporting herbs are available in capsule or tablet form. Make sure to choose supplements that are standardised for their active ingredients (e.g., **silymarin** in milk thistle, **curcumin** in turmeric).

3. **Herbal Tinctures:**

    Tinctures are liquid extracts of herbs and can be added to water, smoothies, or juice. They are an excellent option for those who want a fast-acting herbal solution, as tinctures are absorbed quickly into the bloodstream.

4. **Adding Herbs to Your Cooking:**

    Herbs like **turmeric** and **artichoke** can easily be incorporated into meals. Use turmeric in curries, soups, or smoothies for its liver-protective benefits, and add artichoke to salads or as a side dish to promote healthy digestion and bile flow.

Safety Considerations When Using Herbs

While herbs are natural, they can still interact with medications or have side effects, especially when taken in large doses. Here are a few safety tips to keep in mind:

1. **Consult a Healthcare Provider:**

    Before starting any herbal supplement, it is important to consult with a healthcare provider, especially if you are taking prescription medications. For instance, **milk thistle** may interfere with certain medications metabolised by the liver, and **turmeric** can thin the blood, so it is important to use caution if you're on blood-thinning medications.

2. **Start Slowly:**

    If you're new to herbal supplements, start with a low dose to see how your body reacts. Some people may experience mild digestive upset when taking certain herbs for the first time.

3. **Quality Matters:**

    Choose high-quality herbal supplements from reputable brands. Look for products that are standardised for their active compounds and are free from contaminants like heavy metals and pesticides.

Conclusion

Herbal remedies have been used for centuries to support liver health, and modern research continues to validate their efficacy in promoting detoxification, reducing inflammation, and protecting liver cells from damage. Whether you choose to incorporate **milk thistle, turmeric, dandelion root, schisandra,** or **artichoke leaf** into your routine, these herbs can play a powerful role in maintaining liver health and supporting your body's natural detoxification processes.

By combining traditional knowledge with modern science, you can create a well-rounded approach to liver detoxification that includes both herbal remedies and healthy lifestyle choices. Always remember that while herbs are a valuable tool, they work best when used as part of a holistic approach to liver health, which includes a nutrient-rich diet, regular exercise, and proper hydration.

Chapter Summary

This chapter explored popular herbs for liver detox, including **milk thistle, turmeric, dandelion root, schisandra,** and **artichoke leaf**. Each herb was examined for its liver-protective properties, supported by both traditional uses and modern scientific evidence. We also provided practical guidance on how to incorporate these herbs into your daily routine, along with safety tips for their use. A case history demonstrated how herbal remedies can effectively support liver detox and improve overall health, particularly in cases of mild liver conditions like **NAFLD**.

By embracing the healing power of herbs, you can give your liver the support it needs to function at its best, ensuring long-term health and vitality.

Summary: Herbal and Botanical Support for Liver Detox

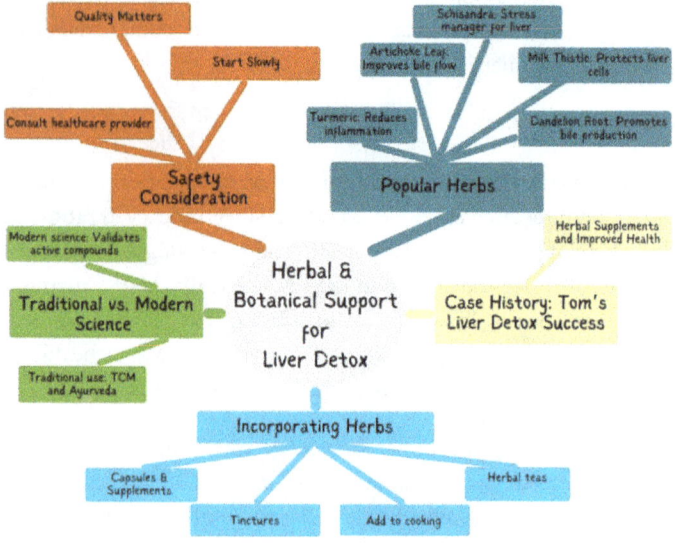

Chapter 6
The Role of Diet in Liver Detox

What we eat plays a crucial role in liver health and its ability to detoxify the body. The liver processes everything we consume, whether it is nutrients or toxins. Therefore, your diet can either support or hinder liver detoxification. In this chapter, we'll explore how specific foods can enhance liver function and detoxification, as well as which foods to avoid that may stress the liver. A well-balanced diet full of liver-friendly foods can dramatically improve your liver's ability to filter out toxins and regenerate.

The Liver's Relationship with Food

The liver is central to digestion and nutrient metabolism. It helps break down fats, carbohydrates, and proteins and stores vital nutrients such as glycogen (stored energy), vitamins, and minerals. When you eat a nutrient-rich diet, your liver is provided with the raw materials it needs to detoxify your body effectively.

However, poor dietary choices—like excessive sugar, trans fats, or alcohol—can overburden the liver, leading to fat accumulation, inflammation, and even liver damage. Let us break down which foods promote liver health and which can harm it.

Anti-Inflammatory Foods for Liver Heal

An anti-inflammatory diet focuses on whole, unprocessed foods rich in antioxidants, vitamins, and minerals. These foods reduce oxidative stress and inflammation in the liver, making it easier for the liver to perform its detoxification functions.

Liver Revival

Leafy Greens and Cruciferous Vegetables

- **Function:**

    Vegetables such as **spinach, kale, broccoli, Brussels sprouts,** and **cauliflower** are rich in **glucosinolates,** sulfur-containing compounds that help activate detoxifying enzymes in the liver. These vegetables support both **Phase 1** and **Phase 2** of liver detoxification by boosting the production of antioxidants and increasing the liver's ability to neutralise toxins.

Analogy: Think of these vegetables as the liver's "fuel," providing it with the essential nutrients it needs to clean out harmful substances and regenerate healthy cells.

- **Scientific Evidence:**

    A study published in *The Journal of Nutrition* showed that diets rich in cruciferous vegetables significantly enhanced the liver's ability to detoxify harmful chemicals, particularly in individuals exposed to environmental toxins. The sulfur-containing compounds found in these vegetables are also linked to improved bile flow, aiding digestion and fat metabolism.

Beets and Carrots

- **Function:**

    Beets and **carrots** are rich in **beta-carotene** and **flavonoids**, which stimulate and support liver function. Beets, in particular, help increase levels of natural detoxifying enzymes such as **glutathione**, which plays a critical role in neutralising free radicals and protecting liver cells from oxidative stress.

Analogy: Beets and carrots act like a turbo boost for the liver's detox machinery, helping it break down toxins faster and more efficiently.

- **Scientific Evidence:**

    Studies have shown that beetroot extract can improve liver function by increasing detoxification enzymes and reducing inflammation. The antioxidant-rich pigments in beets (betacyanins) are particularly effective at protecting the liver from toxin-related damage.

Garlic and Onions

- **Function:**

    Garlic and onions are high in **sulfur** compounds, which are crucial for liver detoxification. Sulfur helps the liver process toxins more efficiently and boosts levels of **glutathione**, the liver's most potent antioxidant.

Analogy: Think of garlic and onions as the liver's cleaning crew—they help scrub away toxins and ensure that the detox pathways remain open and efficient.

- **Scientific Evidence:**

    Research published in *The Journal of Agricultural and Food Chemistry* found that sulfur-containing compounds in garlic, such as **allicin**, can help protect the liver from damage caused by toxins like alcohol and heavy metals.

Healthy Fats and Liver Detox

The liver plays a major role in fat metabolism, breaking down fats into useful energy or storing them for later use. However, consuming the wrong types of fats can lead to fat accumulation in the liver, contributing to conditions like **non-alcoholic fatty liver disease (NAFLD)**. On the other hand, consuming healthy fats can support liver health.

Liver Revival

Healthy Fats: Omega-3 Fatty Acids

- **Function:**

    Omega-3 fatty acids, found in fatty fish like salmon, mackerel, and sardines, as well as flaxseeds and walnuts, have strong anti-inflammatory effects. Omega-3s help reduce fat accumulation in the liver and lower liver inflammation.

Analogy: Omega-3s act like lubrication for the liver, reducing friction (inflammation) and allowing it to function more smoothly.

- **Scientific Evidence:**

    A study published in *The American Journal of Clinical Nutrition* showed that omega-3 fatty acids could reduce liver fat in people with NAFLD, as well as improve liver enzyme levels.

Avocados and Olive Oil

- **Function:**

    Both **avocados** and **olive oil** are rich in **monounsaturated fats**, which support liver health by reducing oxidative stress and inflammation. These healthy fats help balance cholesterol levels, another function controlled by the liver.

Scientific Evidence:

Research has found that olive oil can improve liver enzyme levels and reduce liver fat. A study published in *Liver International* found that daily consumption of olive oil was associated with lower levels of liver fat and improved liver function in people with NAFLD.

Foods to Avoid for Liver Health

While some foods enhance liver detoxification, others place a heavy burden on the liver, leading to fat accumulation, inflammation, and liver damage over time. Here are the main foods to avoid or limit in order to maintain optimal liver function.

Processed Foods

- **Why They're Harmful:**

    Processed foods, especially those high in **trans fats**, **artificial additives**, and **preservatives**, are difficult for the liver to process. They increase oxidative stress and promote inflammation in the liver, contributing to the development of conditions like **NAFLD**.

Analogy: Processed foods are like "junk" clogging up your liver's detox machinery, making it harder for the liver to filter out toxins.

- **Examples:**

    Foods like chips, cookies, fast food, and sugary snacks fall into this category. These foods are often high in refined carbohydrates and hydrogenated oils, which increase fat accumulation in the liver and worsen liver function.

Sugar and Refined Carbohydrates

- **Why They're Harmful:**

    Excess sugar, particularly **fructose**, can overwhelm the liver's ability to metabolise it. When you consume high amounts of sugar, especially in processed forms like soft drinks or desserts, your liver converts the excess into fat, leading to **fatty liver disease**.

Analogy: Consuming too much sugar is like overloading a conveyor belt—the liver can't keep up with processing it, so it starts storing fat.

- **Scientific Evidence:**

    A study in *The Journal of Hepatology* found that high fructose consumption was strongly associated with liver fat accumulation and increased risk of NAFLD. Reducing sugar intake can help reverse fatty liver disease and improve overall liver function.

Alcohol

- **Why It is Harmful:**

    Alcohol is metabolised primarily in the liver, and excessive consumption can overwhelm the liver's detox systems, leading to **alcoholic liver disease, fatty liver**, and ultimately **cirrhosis** if left unchecked. When you drink alcohol, the liver prioritises metabolising it, which can delay the breakdown of other toxins, leading to toxin buildup and liver damage.

Analogy: Alcohol acts like a heavy load on the liver, forcing it to work overtime and causing wear and tear over time.

- **Scientific Evidence:**

    Numerous studies have shown the harmful effects of chronic alcohol consumption on liver health, including the increased risk of fatty liver, inflammation, and cirrhosis. Moderation is key to preventing alcohol-induced liver damage.

Hydration and Liver Health

Staying well-hydrated is crucial for liver detoxification. Water helps flush toxins out of the body and ensures that bile, which aids in digestion and toxin elimination, flows smoothly.

- **Function:**

    Water is essential for every detox process in the body. It helps the liver metabolise fats and carbohydrates, assists in filtering waste, and supports kidney function to excrete toxins. Without enough water, the liver has a harder time flushing out toxins.

- **Recommendation:**

    Aim for at least 8–10 glasses of water per day to stay hydrated and support liver function. Herbal teas like **dandelion root tea** can also be beneficial, as they provide hydration along with liver-supportive herbs.

Case History: Diet and Liver Detox Success Story

Background:

Lisa, a 38-year-old woman, had struggled with digestive issues, fatigue, and brain fog for years. Her blood tests revealed mildly elevated liver enzymes, indicating liver stress. Lisa's diet primarily consisted of processed foods, sugary snacks, and alcohol on the weekends.

The Plan:

Her healthcare provider recommended a liver-friendly diet. Lisa was encouraged to focus on leafy greens, cruciferous vegetables, and healthy fats, particularly omega-3s from fish and plant-based sources like flaxseed and walnuts. She was advised to significantly reduce her intake of processed foods, sugary drinks, and alcohol while increasing her water consumption.

Results:

After three months of adhering to this new diet, Lisa reported significant improvements in her energy levels, digestion, and mental clarity. Her bloating and fatigue diminished, and she was able to think more clearly throughout the day. Follow-up blood tests showed that her liver enzyme levels had returned to normal, indicating a reduction in liver stress. The incorporation of liver-supportive foods and the elimination of harmful dietary elements proved effective in improving her liver function and overall well-being.

Conclusion

The food you eat has a direct and powerful impact on your liver's health and detoxification abilities. Incorporating nutrient-dense, whole foods such as leafy greens, cruciferous vegetables, healthy fats, and antioxidant-rich fruits into your diet can provide the liver with the nutrients it needs to detoxify effectively and repair itself. Conversely, limiting processed foods, sugar, and alcohol can prevent liver overload and reduce the risk of developing fatty liver disease or other liver conditions.

Hydration plays an essential role as well, helping to flush toxins out of the body and support the liver's excretory functions. With the right diet, you can enhance your liver's natural detoxification processes, promote better digestion, and improve your overall health.

Chapter Summary

This chapter examined how diet plays a pivotal role in liver detoxification. Key liver-supportive foods, such as leafy greens, cruciferous vegetables, garlic, and omega-3 fats, help the liver process toxins and reduce inflammation. Conversely, processed foods, excess sugar, and alcohol can overwhelm the liver, leading to fat accumulation and liver damage. The chapter also emphasised the importance of hydration in supporting liver detoxification and provided a case history demonstrating how dietary changes can significantly improve liver function.

By making thoughtful changes to your diet, you can empower your liver to detoxify more efficiently, maintain its health, and support overall well-being.

Liver Revival

Summary: The Role of Diet in Liver Detox

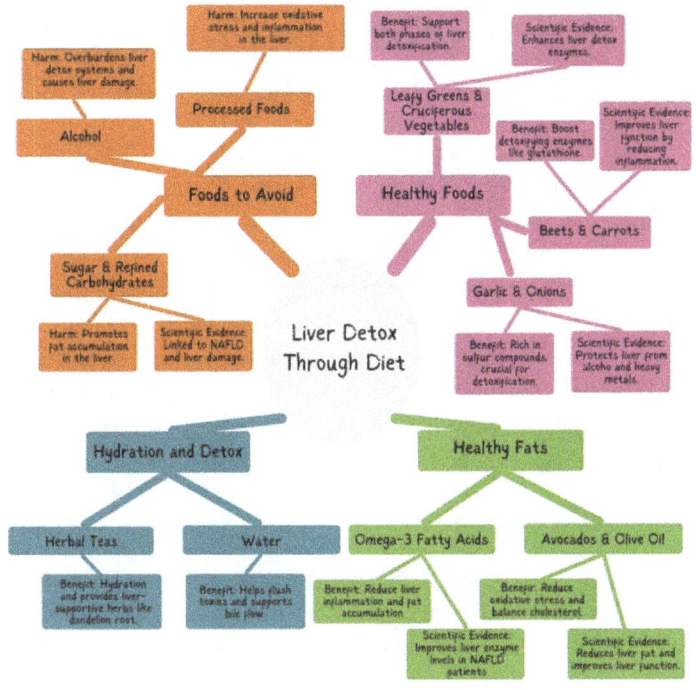

Chapter 7
Fasting and Detoxification: A Powerful Strategy for Liver Health

Fasting, when done correctly, can be one of the most effective methods for enhancing liver detoxification and overall health. By giving the digestive system a break, fasting allows the liver to focus on detoxifying the body, breaking down stored fat, and promoting cellular repair processes like **autophagy**. When combined with the right nutrients and supplements—such as **glutathione, N-acetylcysteine (NAC)**, and **Deliverance**, a new herbal supplement—fasting becomes a safe and powerful strategy for improving liver function and supporting long-term health.

How Fasting Benefits the Liver

Fasting positively impacts the liver in several ways. As the body transitions into a fasting state, it switches from burning glucose (sugar) for energy to burning stored fat. This shift triggers the production of **ketones**, which provide a steady energy source while also reducing inflammation and promoting detoxification.

Glutathione Production

Fasting naturally boosts the production of **glutathione**, the liver's most important antioxidant. Glutathione neutralises free radicals, aids in the detoxification of heavy metals and other toxins, and protects liver cells from damage. When combined with **NAC**—a precursor to glutathione—fasting can enhance the body's ability to produce even higher levels of this essential antioxidant.

- **Analogy**: Glutathione is like the liver's cleaning crew. Fasting gives the crew time to focus without constant interruptions from food intake, allowing them to clean up toxins thoroughly.

- **Scientific Evidence**: Research shows that fasting boosts **glutathione** levels, leading to improved detoxification and liver function. NAC supplementation has been found to increase glutathione production and reduce oxidative stress in the liver.

Fat Burning and Liver Detox

After 12–24 hours of fasting, the liver begins converting stored fat into **ketones** for energy. This fat-burning process helps reduce fat accumulation in the liver, which is especially beneficial for those with **non-alcoholic fatty liver disease (NAFLD)**.

- **Scientific Evidence**: Studies published in *Hepatology* have shown that intermittent fasting can reduce liver fat content and improve liver function in individuals with NAFLD.

Autophagy and Liver Regeneration

Fasting also triggers **autophagy**, a process in which the body breaks down damaged or unnecessary cells and replaces them with new, healthy cells. For the liver, this is particularly beneficial, as it removes damaged liver cells and stimulates the growth of new ones, leading to improved liver function.

- **Analogy**: Autophagy is like the liver's repair crew, clearing out old, damaged cells and rebuilding healthier ones, ensuring the liver functions optimally.

Enhancing Fasting with Glutathione, NAC, and Deliverance

While fasting alone is beneficial for liver detoxification, combining it with specific supplements can amplify its effects. **Glutathione, NAC,** and the new herbal supplement **Deliverance** are powerful tools that can support liver health during fasting.

Liver Revival

Glutathione: The Master Detoxifier

- **Function:**

    Glutathione is the liver's most powerful antioxidant, responsible for neutralising free radicals and aiding in the detoxification of heavy metals and other toxins. Fasting boosts natural glutathione production, but supplementation can provide extra support, particularly during longer fasts.

- **How It Enhances Fasting:**

    Glutathione works synergistically with fasting to boost the liver's detoxification processes. As the liver breaks down fat and releases stored toxins during fasting, glutathione helps neutralise these toxins, ensuring they are safely eliminated from the body.

N-Acetylcysteine (NAC): A Glutathione Precursor

- **Function:**

    NAC is a precursor to glutathione, meaning it helps the body produce more glutathione naturally. NAC also has anti-inflammatory properties, making it particularly useful for individuals with liver inflammation or fatty liver disease.

- **How It Enhances Fasting:**

    By taking NAC during fasting, glutathione levels remain high, allowing the liver to detoxify more efficiently. NAC further reduces inflammation, making it a vital supplement for liver health.

Deliverance: A New Herbal Supplement for Liver Detox

- **Function:**

    Deliverance is a newly developed herbal supplement designed to support liver detox. It contains powerful

53

botanicals like **milk thistle**, **turmeric**, and **schisandra**, known for their liver-protective properties. Deliverance enhances liver function by boosting bile production, improving detoxification, and promoting liver cell regeneration.

- **How It Enhances Fasting:**

    Deliverance helps the liver process and eliminate toxins more efficiently during fasting, while also protecting liver cells from oxidative stress.

Fasting Methods for Liver Detox: A Positive Approach

Intermittent Fasting

Intermittent fasting (IF) is one of the safest and most effective methods for promoting liver detox. With the **16:8 method**, you fast for 16 hours and eat during an 8-hour window. This allows the liver to enter fat-burning mode while maintaining a regular intake of nutrients to support liver function.

- **How to Enhance It:**

    Taking **glutathione** or **NAC** during the fasting period can boost antioxidant levels, while **Deliverance** before meals can enhance bile flow and liver detox.

Extended Fasting (24–48 hours)

Extended fasting can deepen the liver's detox processes by pushing the body into a more pronounced state of ketosis and autophagy. However, it is important to ensure the liver has the nutrients it needs to manage the increased detox load.

- **How to Enhance It:**

    Supplementing with **NAC** and **Deliverance** during extended fasting can provide the liver with extra support, making the detox process more efficient and protecting against oxidative stress.

5:2 Method

The **5:2 method** involves eating normally for five days and restricting calorie intake on two non-consecutive days. This provides the liver with periods of rest and promotes detoxification without requiring prolonged fasting.

- **How to Enhance It:**

    On fasting days, taking **glutathione** or **NAC** can support liver detox, while **Deliverance** throughout the week ensures consistent liver support.

Case History: Fasting with Glutathione, NAC, and Deliver

Background:

Marie, a 42-year-old woman with mild **NAFLD**, felt fatigued and sluggish, with occasional brain fog. After researching fasting, she decided to try intermittent fasting using the **16:8 method**.

The Plan:

Marie began fasting for 16 hours each day and eating during an 8-hour window. She supplemented with **NAC** in the morning to boost glutathione production and took **Deliverance** before meals to support bile flow and liver detox. Her diet focused on whole foods, healthy fats, and cruciferous vegetables.

Results:

After three months, Marie experienced improved energy, digestion, and mental clarity. A follow-up liver ultrasound showed a reduction in liver fat, and her liver enzyme levels had returned to normal. The combination of intermittent fasting, **NAC**, and **Deliverance** provided her liver with the support it needed to detoxify and regenerate.

Conclusion

Fasting, when properly managed, can be one of the most effective ways to detoxify the liver and improve overall health. By boosting natural processes like **glutathione production, fat burning**, and **autophagy**, fasting helps the liver detoxify more efficiently and regenerate healthy cells. When combined with supplements like **glutathione, NAC**, and the herbal supplement **Deliverance**, fasting can become a safe and highly effective strategy for promoting long-term liver health.

Chapter Summary

This chapter highlights how fasting, when done correctly and supported with supplements like **glutathione, NAC,** and **Deliverance**, can be a powerful tool for liver detox. We explored the benefits of fasting for liver function, including promoting autophagy, reducing liver fat, and enhancing detoxification pathways. The chapter also provided practical advice on how to incorporate different fasting methods into your lifestyle, along with a case history that demonstrated the effectiveness of combining fasting with liver-supportive supplements.

Liver Revival

Summary: Fasting and Detoxification: A Powerful Strategy for Liver Health

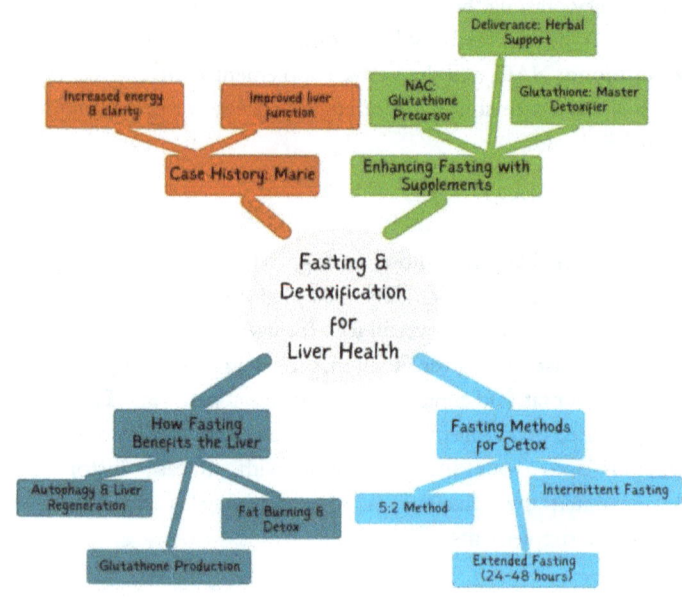

Chapter 8
IV Therapies and Light Therapy for Liver Detox

Modern advancements in medicine have introduced innovative therapies designed to boost liver detoxification and improve overall liver function. Among these therapies, **Intravenous (IV) treatments** and **light therapy** have gained attention for their ability to deliver targeted nutrients and stimulate detoxification processes at a cellular level. These therapies are particularly beneficial for people dealing with liver stress caused by environmental toxins, poor diet, heavy metal exposure, and chronic liver conditions like **non-alcoholic fatty liver disease (NAFLD)** or **hepatitis**.

In this chapter, we'll explore the most effective IV therapies and light treatments for liver detox, including **phosphatidylcholine (PPC), glutathione, alpha-lipoic acid (ALA)**, and **methylene blue**, as well as the benefits of **endolaser light therapy** and **IV Weber Light Therapy**.

IV Therapies for Liver Detox

Intravenous (IV) therapy allows for the direct delivery of nutrients, antioxidants, and medications into the bloodstream. This method bypasses the digestive system, ensuring that the liver receives high concentrations of detoxifying substances that can promote cellular repair and improve overall liver function. Let us look at the key IV therapies commonly used for liver detox:

1. Phosphatidylcholine (PPC)

- **Function:**

    Phosphatidylcholine (PPC) is a key component of cell membranes, particularly in liver cells. It helps repair damaged liver cells, improves bile flow, and reduces inflammation. PPC also plays a role in the metabolism of fats, which is critical for individuals with fatty liver disease or liver congestion.

Analogy: Think of PPC as the "construction material" for the liver's cell walls. When liver cells are damaged by toxins, PPC helps rebuild them, improving the liver's overall structure and function.

- **Scientific Evidence**:

    Several studies have shown that PPC can improve liver enzyme levels and reduce inflammation in patients with liver disease. A clinical study published in *The American Journal of Gastroenterology* found that PPC improved liver function in individuals with chronic liver diseases like **cirrhosis** and **hepatitis**.

- **Benefits for Liver Detox**:

    PPC helps regenerate liver cells, promotes bile flow (critical for detoxification), and aids in the breakdown of fats, making it a valuable therapy for individuals with **NAFLD**, **cholestasis**, or general liver congestion.

2. Glutathione IV Therapy

- **Function**:

    As the liver's most powerful antioxidant, **glutathione** plays a critical role in detoxification. Administering glutathione intravenously ensures high levels of this antioxidant in the bloodstream, which can neutralise free radicals, reduce oxidative stress, and promote liver regeneration.

Analogy: Glutathione is like a detox superhero for the liver, cleaning up toxins and protecting liver cells from damage. IV glutathione gives the liver a concentrated dose of this essential antioxidant, speeding up the detox process.

- **Scientific Evidence:**

    Numerous studies have demonstrated the benefits of glutathione in treating liver conditions. A study published in *Hepatology* found that glutathione improved liver enzyme levels and reduced oxidative damage in individuals with fatty liver disease and other liver conditions.

- **Benefits for Liver Detox:**

    Glutathione IV therapy is especially useful for people exposed to high levels of environmental toxins, heavy metals, or chronic alcohol use. It reduces oxidative stress, promotes detoxification, and helps repair damaged liver cells.

3. Alpha-Lipoic Acid (ALA) IV Therapy

- **Function:**

    Alpha-lipoic acid (ALA) is a potent antioxidant that helps the liver detoxify harmful substances, including heavy metals like mercury and lead. ALA is unique because it is both fat- and water-soluble, meaning it can work in all parts of the liver to reduce oxidative stress and promote cellular repair.

Analogy: ALA is like a versatile cleaning solution that can work in any environment—whether in the fat or water-based parts of the liver—to neutralise toxins and clean up oxidative damage.

- **Scientific Evidence:**

    Studies have shown that ALA can improve liver function and reduce symptoms in patients with liver conditions like **hepatitis C** and **cirrhosis**. Research published in *Liver International* demonstrated that ALA, when administered intravenously, helped reduce liver inflammation and supported the removal of heavy metals from the body.

- **Benefits for Liver Detox:**

    ALA is particularly useful for detoxifying heavy metals and improving liver function in individuals exposed to environmental toxins. It also helps regenerate other antioxidants, such as glutathione, making it a valuable addition to IV liver detox therapies.

4. Methylene Blue IV Therapy

- **Function:**

    Methylene blue is a medication and dye that has been used for decades to treat a variety of conditions. Recently, it has gained attention for its role in promoting mitochondrial function and supporting detoxification. Mitochondria are the energy-producing structures in cells, and improving their function can enhance the liver's ability to process and eliminate toxins.

Analogy: Methylene blue acts like an energy booster for the liver, increasing its efficiency in detoxifying harmful substances by improving cellular energy production.

- **Scientific Evidence:**

    A study published in *Antioxidants & Redox Signaling* found that methylene blue improved mitochondrial function and reduced oxidative stress, which is critical for supporting liver health. By enhancing mitochondrial activity, methylene blue can help the liver detoxify more efficiently.

- **Benefits for Liver Detox:**

    Methylene blue is especially helpful for individuals with chronic fatigue, liver stress, or sluggish detoxification processes. By boosting mitochondrial function, it allows the liver to work more efficiently and detoxify harmful substances faster.

Light Therapy for Liver Detox

Light therapy has become an innovative tool in supporting liver detoxification by stimulating cellular processes through specific wavelengths of light. Two emerging light-based treatments for liver health include **endolaser light therapy** and **IV Weber Light Therapy**.

1. Endolaser Light Therapy

- **Function:**
  Endolaser light therapy involves the use of low-level laser therapy (LLLT) delivered directly to the liver via an intravenous catheter. This therapy stimulates the liver's cells, boosting cellular energy production (via mitochondria) and enhancing detoxification.

Analogy: Think of endolaser therapy as a "power-up" for your liver cells. The laser light energises the liver's detox systems, helping it work more efficiently.

- **Scientific Evidence:**

    Studies show that laser therapy can improve mitochondrial function and reduce inflammation in various tissues, including the liver. A study published in *Lasers in Medical Science* found that low-level laser therapy enhanced cellular repair and detoxification processes in individuals exposed to environmental toxins.

- **Benefits for Liver Detox:**

    Endolaser light therapy helps the liver detoxify more effectively by boosting energy production at the cellular level and promoting faster removal of toxins. It is particularly beneficial for individuals dealing with chronic liver conditions or those exposed to high toxin levels.

2. IV Weber Light Therapy

- **Function:**

    IV Weber Light Therapy is an innovative treatment that delivers specific wavelengths of light (red, green, blue, and yellow) directly into the bloodstream through an intravenous catheter. These light wavelengths help boost detoxification, reduce inflammation, and improve cellular repair by stimulating the body's natural healing processes.

Scientific Evidence:

Research has shown that different wavelengths of light can have various therapeutic effects. For example, **blue light** has strong antibacterial and antiviral properties, while **red light** boosts circulation and cellular repair. A study in *Photomedicine and Laser Surgery* found that IV light therapy can improve blood circulation and enhance detoxification.

- **Benefits for Liver Detox:**

    IV Weber Light Therapy is beneficial for individuals with sluggish detoxification, chronic infections, or liver inflammation. The combination of different light wavelengths helps detoxify the blood and stimulate liver repair processes.

These therapies are particularly beneficial for individuals dealing with toxin overload, chronic liver conditions like **NAFLD**, or those exposed to environmental toxins. The ability to deliver targeted nutrients or light directly into the bloodstream allows for more effective detoxification and cellular repair compared to oral supplementation.

Scientific Backing for IV and Light Therapy

The research behind these treatments supports their efficacy. Studies show that **glutathione** can improve liver function by reducing oxidative stress, while **ALA** helps detoxify heavy metals and regenerate other antioxidants. **Phosphatidylcholine** has been shown to repair liver cells and improve bile flow, crucial for effective detoxification. Moreover, **endolaser light therapy** and **IV Weber Light Therapy** have been found to boost cellular energy, supporting the liver's detoxification capacity.

Case History: Liver Detox with IV Therapy and Light Therapy

Background:

Mike, a 50-year-old man with a history of alcohol use and environmental toxin exposure, had been diagnosed with mild **cirrhosis**. He experienced chronic fatigue, digestive issues, and elevated liver enzymes. Traditional treatments had only provided limited relief, so his doctor recommended IV therapies and light therapy to support liver detoxification and repair.

The Plan:

Mike began a comprehensive detox program that included weekly **IV glutathione** and **alpha-lipoic acid (ALA)** treatments to reduce oxidative stress and promote liver regeneration. He also underwent **endolaser light therapy** sessions twice a month to boost cellular energy and detoxification.

Results:

After three months, Mike's liver enzyme levels had normalised, and he reported improved energy levels and digestion. His doctor noted a significant reduction in liver inflammation and oxidative stress, thanks to the combination of IV therapies and light therapy. Mike continued the treatment regimen to support his liver's long-term health and detox capacity.

Conclusion

IV therapies and light therapy offer powerful, targeted solutions for liver detoxification and repair. These treatments allow the liver to detoxify harmful substances more efficiently while simultaneously regenerating damaged cells and promoting overall health. Whether you are dealing with chronic liver conditions, toxin overload, or simply looking for ways to Optimise liver function, IV therapies such as **glutathione**, **ALA**, and **PPC**, along with **endolaser** and **IV Weber Light Therapy**, provide promising and scientifically-backed approaches to liver health

Summary: IV Therapies and Light Therapy for Liver Detox

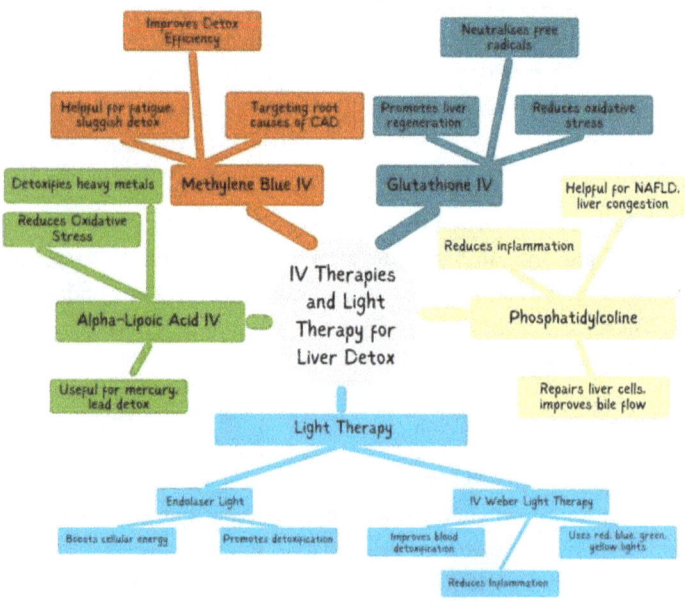

Chapter 9
Heavy Metal Toxicity and Detoxification

Heavy metal toxicity can have serious consequences for liver health, as the liver is the primary organ responsible for filtering and eliminating these harmful substances from the body. Heavy metals such as **mercury, lead, cadmium,** and **arsenic** accumulate in tissues over time, overwhelming the liver's detoxification pathways and contributing to a range of health problems, including **fatigue, neurological issues,** and **liver disease**. In this chapter, we will explore how heavy metals impact the liver, the symptoms of heavy metal toxicity, and the most effective detoxification strategies to help the liver eliminate these toxic substances.

How Heavy Metals Impact the Liver

Heavy metals are persistent in the environment and can enter the body through contaminated food, water, air, or direct exposure in certain occupational settings. Once inside the body, heavy metals bind to proteins and enzymes in the liver, disrupting normal cellular function, damaging liver cells, and impairing the liver's ability to detoxify other substances.

- **Oxidative Stress:**

    Heavy metals generate high levels of **free radicals**—unstable molecules that cause oxidative damage to cells. This oxidative stress overwhelms the liver's antioxidant defences, leading to inflammation and liver cell death.

Analogy: Think of heavy metals as "rust" that accumulates on machinery (liver cells), making it harder for the machinery to function efficiently and causing damage over time.

- **Interference with Enzymes**:

    Heavy metals can inhibit the activity of key liver enzymes involved in detoxification. For example, mercury binds to **selenium**, a mineral required for the function of **glutathione peroxidase**, an important antioxidant enzyme. This interference reduces the liver's ability to neutralise toxins and protect itself from damage.

- **Bile Production**:

    Heavy metals can also disrupt bile production and flow. Bile is essential for the elimination of fat-soluble toxins, so impaired bile flow leads to the accumulation of these toxins in the liver and other tissues.

Symptoms of Heavy Metal Toxicity

Heavy metal toxicity can present with a wide range of symptoms, depending on the specific metal involved and the degree of exposure. Common symptoms include:

- **Fatigue**: Chronic exposure to heavy metals can cause persistent fatigue, as the body struggles to detoxify and eliminate the metals.

- **Cognitive Dysfunction**: Memory loss, brain fog, and difficulty concentrating are often reported in individuals with high levels of heavy metals, as these toxins can accumulate in the brain and disrupt normal neurological function.

- **Digestive Issues**: Heavy metals can impair liver function, leading to symptoms like **bloating**, **constipation**, and **poor digestion**.

- **Skin Problems**: Heavy metal toxicity can manifest as skin rashes, acne, or eczema, as the liver's reduced detox capacity causes toxins to be eliminated through the skin.

- **Immune Dysfunction**: Heavy metals can weaken the immune system, leading to increased susceptibility to infections and autoimmune conditions.

Oligoscan Testing for Heavy Metal Toxicity

Oligoscan testing is a non-invasive diagnostic tool that measures the levels of heavy metals and trace elements in the body by analyzing the skin. This test can provide valuable information about an individual's exposure to heavy metals and can guide personalised detoxification strategies.

- **How It Works**:

    Oligoscan uses a technology called **spectrophotometry** to analyze the light reflected from the skin, providing real-time data on the concentration of heavy metals like mercury, lead, cadmium, and aluminium. The test is painless and takes only a few minutes.

- **Benefits**:

    Oligoscan testing offers a quick and convenient way to assess heavy metal toxicity without the need for invasive blood tests or urine analysis. It provides immediate results, allowing healthcare providers to create targeted detoxification protocols based on the specific metals detected.

Case Example:

Jane, a 45-year-old woman, experienced chronic fatigue, headaches, and digestive issues. After undergoing an Oligoscan test, high levels of mercury and cadmium were detected. Her doctor recommended a heavy metal detox program, which included chelation therapy, dietary changes, and antioxidant supplementation.

Liver Revival

Strategies for Heavy Metal Detoxification

Once heavy metal toxicity has been identified, detoxification strategies focus on supporting the liver and kidneys in eliminating these toxic substances from the body. Here are the most effective methods for detoxifying heavy metals:

1. Chelation Therapy

- **Function:**

    Chelation therapy involves the use of specific compounds, known as **chelating agents**, that bind to heavy metals in the bloodstream and allow them to be excreted through the urine. Chelating agents include **EDTA (ethylenediaminetetraacetic acid), DMSA (Dimercaptosuccinic acid),** and **DMPS (Dimercaptopropane sulfonate).**

Analogy: Chelating agents act like magnets, attracting heavy metals and pulling them out of the body through urine.

- **Scientific Evidence:**

    Numerous studies have demonstrated the effectiveness of chelation therapy in treating heavy metal poisoning. A study published in *Environmental Health Perspectives* found that chelation therapy significantly reduced blood levels of lead and improved symptoms in individuals with lead poisoning.

- **Application:**

    Chelation therapy is typically administered under the supervision of a healthcare provider and can be given intravenously or orally, depending on the specific agent used.

2. Glutathione and NAC for Heavy Metal Detox

- **Function:**

    Glutathione is a powerful antioxidant that binds to heavy metals and helps neutralise them so they can be excreted by the liver. **N-acetylcysteine (NAC)** is a precursor to glutathione and helps boost glutathione levels in the liver.

How It Works:

Glutathione and NAC protect liver cells from oxidative damage caused by heavy metals and support the liver's detoxification pathways. Supplementing with glutathione or NAC can be particularly helpful for individuals with high levels of mercury or arsenic.

Scientific Evidence:

Research published in *The Journal of Toxicology* found that glutathione levels were significantly depleted in individuals with heavy metal exposure, and supplementation helped restore liver function and reduce oxidative stress.

3. Alpha-Lipoic Acid (ALA)

- **Function:**

    Alpha-lipoic acid (ALA) is a potent antioxidant that plays a key role in detoxifying heavy metals, particularly mercury. ALA is unique in that it can cross the blood-brain barrier, helping remove heavy metals from both the liver and the brain.

Scientific Evidence:

Studies have shown that ALA can bind to heavy metals and enhance their excretion from the body. Research published in *Free Radical Biology and Medicine* found that ALA reduced mercury levels in individuals exposed to the metal.

Benefits:

ALA not only helps detoxify heavy metals but also regenerates other antioxidants, such as glutathione, which further enhances detoxification.

4. The Role of Diet in Heavy Metal Detox

Dietary changes can play a significant role in supporting the liver's ability to detoxify heavy metals. Consuming nutrient-rich, detox-supportive foods can enhance the body's natural detoxification processes and reduce the burden on the liver.

- **Cruciferous Vegetables:**

    Vegetables like **broccoli, Brussels sprouts**, and **kale** are rich in sulfur-containing compounds that support liver detoxification enzymes and help neutralise heavy metals.

- **Cilantro:**

    Cilantro is known for its ability to bind to heavy metals, particularly mercury, and assist in their elimination from the body. Adding cilantro to your diet can support the liver's detox efforts.

- **Chlorella:**

    Chlorella is a type of green algae that binds to heavy metals and promotes their excretion. It is often used in conjunction with cilantro to enhance the removal of heavy metals from the body.

Case History: Detoxing from Mercury Exposure

Background:

Tom, a 52-year-old man, worked in a dental office for years and was exposed to **mercury** from dental amalgam fillings. He began experiencing symptoms such as brain fog, fatigue, and muscle weakness. After an Oligoscan test revealed high mercury levels, Tom's doctor recommended a comprehensive detox program.

The Plan:

Tom underwent **chelation therapy** with **DMPS**, along with regular IV **glutathione** treatments to support his liver's detox pathways. He also took **NAC** and **ALA** to boost antioxidant levels and help detoxify his liver and brain. In addition, Tom incorporated **cilantro** and **chlorella** into his diet to further assist with mercury elimination.

Results:

After six months, Tom's mercury levels had significantly decreased, and he reported improvements in his energy, mental clarity, and muscle strength. Follow-up tests showed that his liver function had improved, and he continued to use cilantro and chlorella to support ongoing detoxification.

Conclusion

Heavy metal toxicity poses a significant challenge to liver health, but with the right detoxification strategies, the liver can effectively eliminate these harmful substances from the body. **Chelation therapy, glutathione, NAC, ALA,** and targeted dietary changes provide powerful tools to support liver detoxification and protect the body from the damaging effects of heavy metals.

Whether dealing with acute heavy metal poisoning or chronic exposure, addressing heavy metal toxicity is crucial for preventing long-term health problems. Using diagnostic tools like **Oligoscan testing** allows for personalised detoxification plans, ensuring that individuals receive the most effective treatments for their specific toxicity levels. A combination of medical interventions like **chelation therapy** and natural strategies like **cilantro** and **chlorella** can help restore optimal liver function and reduce the burden of heavy metal accumulation.

Liver Revival

Summary: Heavy Metal Toxicity and Detoxification

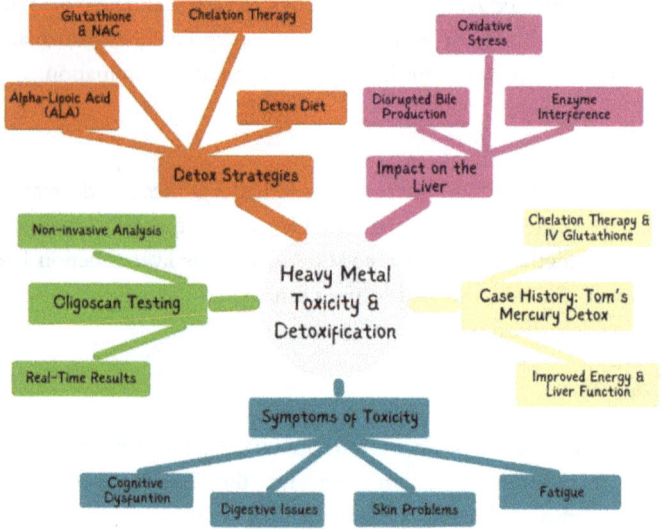

Chapter 10
Liver Detox for Children

When we think about liver detoxification, we often associate it with adults, particularly those exposed to environmental toxins, processed foods, or alcohol. However, children are also susceptible to liver-related issues, albeit for different reasons. Their growing bodies may be more vulnerable to toxins from the environment, food, medications, and other sources. The liver plays a crucial role in detoxifying these substances, but when overloaded, it can lead to health problems that affect both physical and cognitive development.

In this chapter, we'll explore the unique considerations for liver detox in children, safe and effective detox methods, and how to support liver health through nutrition and gentle detox practices.

Why Children Need Liver Detox Support

Children's bodies are in a constant state of growth and development, and their organs, including the liver, are still maturing. While the liver in a child functions similarly to an adult's liver in detoxifying harmful substances, it may not always have the same resilience or capacity to cope with large toxin loads.

Toxin Exposure in Children

Some of the most common sources of toxins for children include:

- **Environmental Toxins**:

    Children are exposed to various environmental toxins from air pollution, pesticides in food, and heavy metals such as lead and mercury. These toxins can accumulate in the liver, making it harder for the organ to detoxify properly.

- **Medications**:

    Certain medications prescribed during childhood, particularly those for chronic conditions or infections, can place stress on the liver. For example, prolonged use of antibiotics or acetaminophen (a common pain reliever) can overburden the liver's detox pathways.

- **Processed Foods**:

    Many processed foods targeted at children contain additives, preservatives, and high levels of sugar, all of which can contribute to liver congestion. Regular consumption of these foods can lead to the accumulation of toxins and may affect liver function.

- **Household Products and Chemicals**:

    Children are often exposed to chemicals found in household cleaning products, plastic toys, and personal care products. Over time, these substances can build up in the body and place an added burden on the liver.

Symptoms of Liver Stress in Children

The liver performs many vital functions, including detoxification, digestion, and nutrient storage. When the liver is under stress, children may experience a variety of symptoms, including:

- **Fatigue**: Chronic tiredness or lack of energy may indicate liver overload.

- **Skin Problems**: Rashes, eczema, and acne may be signs that the liver is struggling to eliminate toxins.

- **Digestive Issues**: Bloating, constipation, or frequent digestive discomfort may occur when the liver's detox pathways are congested.

- **Behavioural Changes**: Mood swings, irritability, or difficulty concentrating can sometimes result from toxin accumulation affecting brain function.

Safe Detox Solutions for Children

Because children's bodies are still developing, any detoxification process needs to be gentle and carefully managed. Below are some safe and effective methods to support liver detox in children.

1. Nutrient-dense diet for Liver Health

The foundation of any liver detox program for children should be a diet rich in nutrients that support the liver's natural detoxification processes. Key elements include:

- **Leafy Greens**: Spinach, kale, and other greens contain **chlorophyll**, which helps cleanse the liver and support detoxification pathways. These vegetables also provide antioxidants that protect liver cells from damage.

- **Cruciferous Vegetables**: Broccoli, cauliflower, and Brussels sprouts are rich in **sulfur compounds**, which help boost liver enzyme activity, aiding in detoxification. These vegetables also promote bile production, which helps the liver remove toxins.

- **Berries and Citrus Fruits**: Berries, oranges, and lemons are packed with antioxidants, such as **vitamin C**, which helps the liver neutralise free radicals and improve the detoxification process.

- **Healthy Fats**: Avocados, olive oil, and nuts provide essential fatty acids that support the liver's ability to metabolise fats and reduce inflammation.

- **Hydration**: Drinking plenty of water is essential for supporting liver detoxification, as it helps flush toxins from the body. Encourage children to drink water throughout the day and limit sugary drinks that can overburden the liver.

2. Gentle Herbal Support

Some herbs are known for their gentle liver detox properties and can be safely used with children under the guidance of a healthcare provider. Examples include:

- **Milk Thistle (Silybum marianum):**

    Milk thistle is one of the most well-known liver-protective herbs. Its active compound, **silymarin**, helps protect liver cells from damage, supports liver regeneration, and boosts antioxidant production. Although commonly used in adults, milk thistle can also be used in small, carefully monitored doses for children.

- **Dandelion Root (Taraxacum officinale):**

    Dandelion root stimulates bile production and supports the liver's ability to detoxify fat-soluble toxins. It also acts as a mild diuretic, helping flush toxins through the kidneys.

- **Turmeric (Curcuma longa):**

    Turmeric contains **curcumin**, a compound known for its powerful anti-inflammatory and antioxidant properties. It helps reduce liver inflammation and supports detoxification. Curcumin supplements designed for children can be a safe addition to a liver detox program.

3. Supporting Digestive Health

Since the liver and digestive system are closely linked, it is important to support digestion during a detox program. Healthy digestion ensures that toxins are eliminated efficiently and don't recirculate in the body.

- **Fibre-Rich Foods:**

    Foods high in fibre, such as oats, apples, and sweet potatoes, can help bind toxins in the digestive tract and promote their excretion through the bowels.

- **Probiotics:**

    Gut health plays a significant role in liver function, as beneficial gut bacteria aid in the breakdown and elimination of toxins. Probiotic supplements or fermented foods like yoghurt and kefir can support a healthy gut microbiome in children.

Detox Practices for Children

In addition to dietary and herbal support, there are some gentle detox practices that can help reduce toxin load and support liver health in children.

1. Limiting Toxin Exposure

Reducing children's exposure to toxins is an important step in liver detox. This can be done by:

- Choosing organic produce when possible to reduce pesticide exposure.
- Using non-toxic cleaning products and personal care items.
- Limiting plastic use, especially plastic food containers and water bottles that may contain harmful chemicals like BPA (bisphenol A).

2. Movement and Exercise

Regular physical activity supports liver detoxification by improving circulation and encouraging the movement of lymphatic fluid, which helps remove toxins from the body. Encourage outdoor play and age-appropriate physical activities that children enjoy.

3. Adequate Sleep

The liver carries out many of its detoxification processes while the body is at rest, particularly during deep sleep. Ensuring that children get adequate, quality sleep is critical for supporting liver health and overall well-being. Establishing a regular sleep routine can help promote better sleep patterns and support detoxification.

Case History: Liver Detox in a Child with Eczema

Background:

Emily, a 7-year-old girl, had been suffering from eczema for two years. Her parents had tried various creams and medications with limited success. Emily also experienced occasional digestive discomfort and frequent colds, suggesting her immune system was under strain. A holistic healthcare provider suggested that her liver might be struggling to detoxify efficiently, leading to her skin issues.

The Plan:

Emily's healthcare provider recommended a gentle liver detox program that focused on improving her diet, adding liver-supportive herbs, and addressing her gut health. Emily's diet was rich in leafy greens, cruciferous vegetables, berries, and healthy fats. She was given a mild milk thistle tincture to support liver function and a probiotic supplement to improve her gut health.

Results:

Within three months, Emily's eczema had improved significantly. Her digestion also became more regular, and she had fewer colds. Her parents noticed that her energy levels were higher, and she was less irritable. Emily continued to follow the liver-supportive diet, and her symptoms remained under control.

Conclusion

Supporting liver detox in children is an important aspect of maintaining their overall health and well-being. By focusing on nutrient-dense foods, gentle herbal support, and healthy lifestyle practices, we can help reduce the toxin load on the liver and promote efficient detoxification. While children are resilient, their growing bodies need support to cope with environmental toxins, medications, and modern dietary habits.

A balanced approach to liver detoxification, emphasising nutrition, gentle supplements, and healthy habits, can help ensure that children's livers are functioning optimally, allowing them to thrive physically and mentally.

Chapter Summary

This chapter explored the importance of liver detox for children, highlighting the unique challenges they face from environmental toxins, medications, and processed foods. It outlined safe and effective detox strategies, including nutrient-rich diets, gentle herbal support, probiotics, and lifestyle changes. A real-life case history demonstrated the effectiveness of these strategies in addressing liver overload and improving symptoms like eczema and digestive issues.

Liver Revival

Summary: Liver Detox for Children

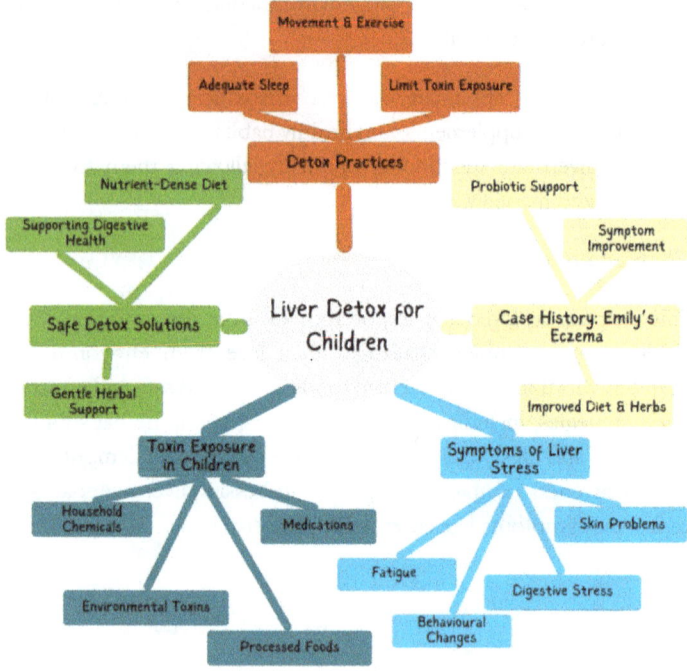

Chapter 11
Ancient Practices in Liver Health

The concept of liver detoxification is not a modern invention. For thousands of years, various ancient medical systems have emphasised the importance of liver health as central to overall well-being. From **Traditional Chinese Medicine (TCM)** to **Ayurveda** and **Ancient Greek Medicine**, these ancient healing systems offer valuable insights into the maintenance of liver health. Interestingly, many of their practices and herbal remedies for liver detoxification have been validated by modern science, demonstrating their enduring relevance.

In this chapter, we'll explore the ancient approaches to liver health, the herbs and practices that were used, and how these traditional methods can be incorporated into modern liver detox protocols.

Traditional Chinese Medicine (TCM) and Liver Detox

In **Traditional Chinese Medicine (TCM)**, the liver is considered the organ responsible for maintaining the smooth flow of **Qi (vital energy)** throughout the body. TCM sees the liver as playing a central role in emotional regulation, blood storage, and detoxification. The liver in TCM is linked to the element of wood and is believed to play a key role in managing the body's emotional and physical balance.

The Liver's Functions in TCM

1. **Regulation of Qi:**

    In TCM, the liver is responsible for maintaining the smooth flow of Qi. If the liver's Qi becomes stagnant, symptoms like irritability, frustration, and digestive problems can arise. Liver Qi stagnation is a common diagnosis in TCM for those experiencing stress or emotional tension.

2. **Blood Storage and Detoxification:**

> The liver stores blood and helps regulate its movement. It also aids in detoxification by filtering impurities and supporting the natural elimination of toxins. Liver detox in TCM is often tied to blood purification, making the liver essential in preventing toxic buildup.

Herbs for Liver Detox in TCM

Several key herbs have been used in TCM for centuries to promote liver health and detoxification. These include:

- **Bupleurum (Chai Hu):**

> Known for its ability to regulate liver Qi, bupleurum is used to relieve liver stagnation and emotional tension. It is a common ingredient in TCM formulas designed to support liver function.

- **Schisandra (Wu Wei Zi):**

> Schisandra berries are known to support the liver's detoxification pathways by enhancing antioxidant activity and protecting liver cells. This adaptogen herb also strengthens the liver's energy or Qi.

- **Chinese Skullcap (Huang Qin):**

> This herb has anti-inflammatory and liver-protective properties, making it a popular choice in TCM for treating liver conditions like hepatitis or liver inflammation.

TCM Liver Detox Practices

In addition to herbal remedies, TCM employs therapies like **acupuncture** to stimulate the liver meridian and restore the flow of Qi. TCM practitioners often recommend acupuncture treatments to address liver stagnation, emotional imbalances and to promote detoxification.

Liver Revival

Ayurveda and Liver Health

In **Ayurveda**, the liver is seen as a key organ involved in digestion and detoxification. Ayurveda emphasises the role of the liver in balancing the body's **Agni (digestive fire)** and purifying **Rakta dhatu (blood)**. Liver health in Ayurveda is closely linked to the balance of the three doshas: **Vata**, **Pitta**, and **Kapha**.

The Liver and Pitta Dosha

In Ayurveda, the liver is most closely associated with the **Pitta dosha**, which governs metabolism, digestion, and transformation. Imbalances in Pitta often manifest as liver dysfunction, leading to symptoms like inflammation, indigestion, and excess heat in the body.

Ayurvedic Herbs for Liver Detox

Ayurvedic texts provide detailed instructions on herbal treatments that support liver detoxification. Some of the most effective herbs include:

- **Turmeric (Haridra):**

    Turmeric is well-known in both Ayurveda and modern medicine for its potent anti-inflammatory and antioxidant properties. It helps reduce liver inflammation, promotes bile production, and supports the liver's natural detoxification processes.

- **Guduchi (Tinospora cordifolia):**

    Known as a rejuvenating herb, Guduchi is commonly used in Ayurveda to treat liver disorders. It strengthens the immune system, detoxifies the liver, and reduces inflammation.

- **Kutki (Picrorhiza kurroa):**

    Kutki is an Ayurvedic herb with strong hepatoprotective properties. It helps treat liver conditions like jaundice and fatty liver disease by stimulating bile production and improving liver function.

Ayurvedic Detox Practices

Ayurvedic liver detox is often part of a holistic cleansing program like **Panchakarma**, which includes:

- **Abhyanga (Oil Massage):**

    This daily oil massage is used to stimulate lymphatic drainage, improve circulation, and support the removal of toxins from the body.

- **Basti (Herbal Enemas):**

    Basti treatments use medicated enemas to cleanse the colon and promote the elimination of toxins, supporting the liver's detoxification role.

- **Diet and Fasting:**

    Ayurveda recommends light diets and occasional fasting to support digestion and allow the liver to focus on detoxifying the body.

Ancient Greek Medicine and the Liver

In **Ancient Greek Medicine**, the liver was viewed as one of the body's most vital organs. **Hippocrates**, often called the "Father of Medicine," described the liver as the body's central organ for digestion and detoxification. The Greeks believed that the liver regulated the body's vital fluids, including bile and blood, and played a key role in maintaining health.

Greek Herbs for Liver Health

The ancient Greeks used several herbs to support liver health and detoxification. Many of these remedies are still used in modern herbal medicine:

- **Milk Thistle (Silybum marianum):**

    Milk thistle has been used since ancient times for its liver-protective properties. The active compound **silymarin** supports liver cell regeneration and protects the liver from damage caused by toxins.

- **Dandelion (Taraxacum officinale):**

    Dandelion root was used by the ancient Greeks to support digestion and liver detox. Dandelion stimulates bile production, helping the liver remove toxins more efficiently.

- **Artichoke (Cynara scolymus):**

    Artichoke was valued by the ancient Greeks for its ability to stimulate bile flow and protect liver cells from oxidative stress.

Fasting and Detox Practices

The Greeks frequently practised fasting as a means of cleansing the liver and improving digestion. Fasting allowed the body to focus on eliminating toxins, and it was believed to "reset" the digestive system. Additionally, the use of bitter herbs to stimulate liver function was a common practice in Ancient Greek Medicine.

Modern Science Meets Ancient Wisdom

Many of the ancient liver detox practices from TCM, Ayurveda, and Greek medicine have been validated by modern science. For example:

- **Milk Thistle:** Modern research shows that silymarin from milk thistle has strong antioxidant and hepatoprotective effects, supporting liver detoxification and reducing inflammation.

- **Turmeric**: Studies confirm turmeric's ability to enhance bile production, reduce liver inflammation, and protect liver cells from damage.

- **Schisandra**: Research supports schisandra's role in increasing antioxidant activity in the liver, promoting detoxification and protecting against oxidative damage.

Case Study:

John, a 45-year-old man, experienced chronic fatigue, bloating, and mild liver inflammation. He consulted a holistic practitioner who recommended an Ayurvedic detox protocol, including turmeric and Guduchi. After following the detox plan for six weeks, John's liver enzymes returned to normal, and his symptoms significantly improved.

Conclusion

Ancient practices for liver health, as seen in **Traditional Chinese Medicine, Ayurveda,** and **Ancient Greek Medicine,** offer timeless wisdom that can be integrated into modern detox protocols. These systems emphasise balance, purification, and the use of herbs to support the liver's detoxification processes. Today, we can combine this ancient wisdom with modern science to create holistic and effective liver detox strategies that promote long-term health and vitality.

Chapter Summary

This chapter explored traditional approaches to liver health from **Traditional Chinese Medicine, Ayurveda,** and **Ancient Greek Medicine**. Each system offers unique insights into detoxification through the use of herbs, dietary practices, and lifestyle modifications. Modern science has validated many of these ancient approaches, highlighting their continued relevance in supporting liver detoxification today.

Summary: *Ancient Practices in Liver Health*

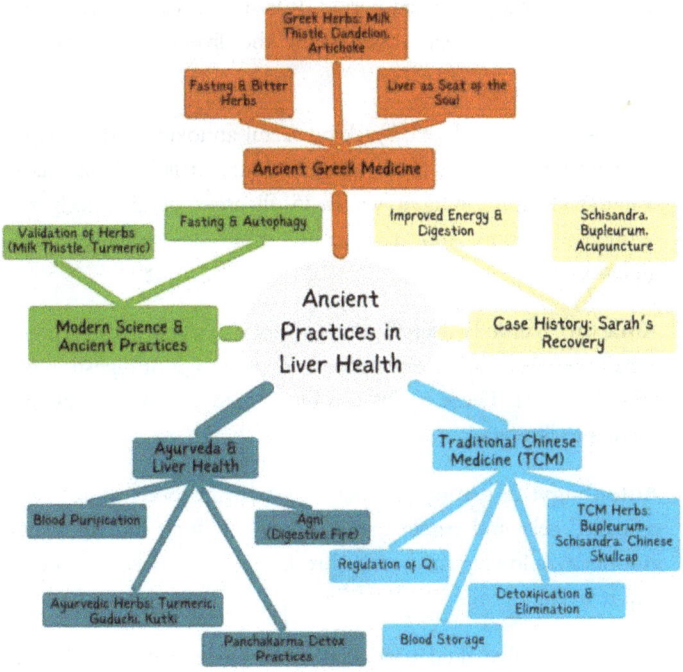

Glossary

1. **Acetaminophen**: A common over-the-counter pain reliever and fever reducer that can cause liver damage when taken in large doses or over a prolonged period. It is metabolised in the liver, and excessive use can overwhelm the liver's detoxification pathways.

2. **Alpha-Lipoic Acid (ALA)**: A powerful antioxidant that helps detoxify heavy metals, particularly mercury. It is both fat- and water-soluble, meaning it works in all areas of the body to neutralise toxins and regenerate other antioxidants, like glutathione.

3. **Ama**: In Ayurveda, "ama" refers to toxic waste or undigested substances that accumulate in the body due to poor digestion or lifestyle habits. These toxins can block natural detox pathways, leading to illness.

4. **Autophagy**: A natural process by which the body cleans out damaged cells and regenerates new ones. Fasting can stimulate autophagy, allowing the liver to break down harmful substances and rejuvenate.

5. **Bile**: A digestive fluid produced by the liver that helps break down fats into fatty acids. It also plays a key role in removing waste products from the liver and aiding in the elimination of toxins through the digestive system.

6. **Chelation Therapy**: A medical treatment that uses chelating agents, such as EDTA or DMPS, to bind to heavy metals in the body, allowing them to be safely excreted. It is often used to treat heavy metal poisoning and to detoxify the liver.

7. **Cirrhosis**: A chronic liver disease characterised by the replacement of healthy liver tissue with scar tissue, often as a result of long-term damage from alcohol, hepatitis, or other

causes. Cirrhosis impairs liver function and its ability to detoxify the body.

8. **Cytokines**: Small proteins released by cells that have an effect on the interactions and communications between cells. High levels of inflammatory cytokines can be produced in response to liver inflammation, contributing to liver damage and disease.

9. **Detoxification**: The liver's natural process of breaking down and removing harmful substances from the body, including toxins, chemicals, and waste products. Detoxification occurs in two phases (Phase 1 and Phase 2) and requires nutrients, antioxidants, and enzymes to function efficiently.

10. **Fatty Liver Disease**: A condition where excess fat builds up in the liver cells. It can be caused by alcohol consumption (alcoholic fatty liver disease) or other factors like poor diet and obesity (non-alcoholic fatty liver disease, NAFLD). Fatty liver can lead to inflammation and liver damage over time.

11. **Glutathione**: A powerful antioxidant produced naturally by the liver. It plays a critical role in detoxification by neutralising free radicals, protecting liver cells, and supporting the elimination of toxins. Glutathione levels can be boosted through supplementation with N-acetylcysteine (NAC).

12. **Hepatoprotective**: Refers to substances that protect the liver from damage. Many herbs and compounds, such as milk thistle and turmeric, are considered hepatoprotective because they help prevent liver injury and support regeneration.

13. **Jaundice**: A condition characterised by yellowing of the skin and eyes due to high levels of bilirubin in the blood. It is often a sign of liver dysfunction or bile duct blockage, as the liver is responsible for processing and eliminating bilirubin.

14. **Liver Enzymes (ALT, AST)**: Enzymes produced by the liver that help facilitate various metabolic processes. Elevated levels of liver enzymes in the blood can indicate liver inflammation or

damage, which may result from conditions like fatty liver disease, hepatitis, or toxin overload.

15. **Milk Thistle (Silybum marianum):** An herb widely used for its liver-protective properties. The active compound, silymarin, helps protect liver cells from toxins, promotes regeneration, and supports overall liver function.

16. **N-Acetylcysteine (NAC):** A supplement that serves as a precursor to glutathione, helping the liver produce more of this critical antioxidant. NAC is often used in liver detox protocols to protect against oxidative stress and support the detoxification of toxins.

17. **Non-Alcoholic Fatty Liver Disease (NAFLD):** A liver condition characterised by the accumulation of fat in liver cells not caused by alcohol consumption. It is closely associated with obesity, insulin resistance, and metabolic syndrome and can progress to more severe liver diseases like non-alcoholic steatohepatitis (NASH).

18. **Oligoscan:** A non-invasive diagnostic tool used to measure heavy metals and trace elements in the body by analyzing the light reflected off the skin. Oligoscan results help healthcare providers design personalised detoxification plans based on heavy metal toxicity levels.

19. **Panchakarma:** A detoxification and rejuvenation program used in Ayurveda that involves five therapeutic procedures to eliminate toxins from the body, cleanse the organs, and restore balance to the body's doshas. Panchakarma often includes therapies like oil massage, steam baths, and herbal enemas.

20. **Phosphatidylcholine (PPC):** A key component of cell membranes, particularly in liver cells. PPC helps repair damaged liver cells, improves bile flow, and supports the metabolism of fats, making it beneficial for conditions like fatty liver disease.

21. **Silymarin**: The active compound in milk thistle that is known for its antioxidant and hepatoprotective effects. Silymarin helps protect liver cells from toxins, supports regeneration, and enhances the liver's detoxification capacity.

22. **Toxins**: Harmful substances that enter the body through food, air, water, or direct contact. Toxins can come from environmental pollutants, medications, processed foods, and heavy metals. The liver plays a critical role in detoxifying and eliminating these toxins from the body.

23. **Turmeric (Curcuma longa)**: A spice widely used for its anti-inflammatory and antioxidant properties. The active compound, curcumin, has been shown to reduce liver inflammation, promote bile production, and support liver detoxification processes.

24. **Phase 1 and Phase 2 Detoxification**: The two main phases of liver detoxification. **Phase 1** involves the oxidation of toxins to make them water-soluble, while **Phase 2** involves conjugating these toxins with molecules like glutathione to make them easier to excrete. Both phases require adequate nutrients and enzymes to function properly.

References

Books and Textbooks

1. "The Detox Miracle Sourcebook" by Robert Morse, N.D.

    Focuses on natural detox methods, including liver detoxification, and offers insight into the role of herbs.

2. "The Liver Cleansing Diet" by Dr. Sandra Cabot

    A popular book offering dietary recommendations for liver health and detoxification.

3. **"Fatty Liver: You Can Reverse It"** by Sandra Cabot and Thomas Eanelli

    Provides insights into fatty liver disease, its causes, and effective detox strategies.

4. "Clean: The Revolutionary Program to Restore the Body's Natural Ability to Heal Itself" by Alejandro Junger, M.D.

    A guide to detoxification and cleansing, including liver detox protocols.

5. "Detoxification and Healing" by Sidney Baker, M.D.

    Covers the science behind detoxification and its therapeutic effects on the liver and other organs.

6. **"The Detox Solution"** by Patricia Fitzgerald

    Discusses detox programs for liver health, focusing on nutrition, supplements, and lifestyle changes.

7. **"The Encyclopedia of Natural Medicine"** by Michael Murray, N.D. and Joseph Pizzorno, N.D.

Comprehensive resource on natural treatments, including liver detox strategies.

8. "The Fourfold Path to Healing" by Thomas S. Cowan, M.D.

    Integrates ancient traditions like Ayurveda with modern approaches to liver detox and health.

9. "The Detox Diet: The Definitive Guide for Lifelong Vitality" by Elson M. Haas, M.D.

    Includes protocols for liver detoxification through diet and supplementation.

10. "Herbal Medicine: Biomolecular and Clinical Aspects" by Iris F. F. Benzie and Sissi Wachtel-Galor

    Discusses the pharmacology of various herbs used for liver detox, including milk thistle and dandelion.

11. "Functional Medicine: A Systems Approach to Reversing the Epidemic of Chronic Disease" by Dr. Jeffrey Bland

    Provides a deep dive into detox pathways and liver support.

12. **"The Textbook of Functional Medicine"** by The Institute for Functional Medicine

    Explores the liver's role in detoxification and overall health through a functional medicine perspective.

Scientific Research Papers and Journal Articles

13. **"The Liver as an Organ of Detoxification"** by K.J. Ishak (2020), *Clinical Liver Disease*

    Discusses the liver's role in detoxifying environmental toxins and heavy metals.

14. "Mechanisms of Liver Regeneration and Repair" by Michalopoulos and DeFrances (2005), *Science*

Explores liver regeneration and how detox processes support it.

15. "The Role of Glutathione in the Liver Detoxification" by Dringen et al. (2000), *Journal of Neurochemistry*

    Reviews the function of glutathione in liver detoxification.

16. "Nutritional and Herbal Supplements for Liver Detoxification" by Pradeep Kumar et al. (2018), *Journal of Hepatology*

    Reviews herbs and supplements that support liver detox.

17. "Silymarin and Its Role in Liver Disease: A Review" by Flora et al. (1998), *Phytotherapy Research*

    Discusses the liver-protective effects of milk thistle.

18. **"Alpha-Lipoic Acid as a Hepatoprotective Antioxidant"** by Packer et al. (1995), *Free Radical Biology and Medicine*
    Examines ALA's role in reducing liver oxidative stress.

19. **"The Protective Effects of NAC on Liver Function"** by Ahlfors et al. (2000), *The Journal of Clinical Investigation*
    Highlights the importance of NAC in liver health.

20. **"Endogenous Detoxification Pathways: The Role of Diet and Lifestyle"** by Lambert and Brandt (2013), *Journal of Nutrition and Metabolism*
    Focuses on dietary and lifestyle interventions for supporting liver detox.

21. **"Heavy Metal Toxicity and Liver Health"** by Risher and Amler (2005), *Environmental Health Perspectives*
    Reviews the impact of heavy metals on liver function and detox pathways.

22. **"Non-Alcoholic Fatty Liver Disease (NAFLD) and Liver Detoxification"** by Byrne et al. (2010), *Journal of Hepatology*
    Discusses how diet and lifestyle changes impact liver detox in NAFLD.

23. **"Bupleurum and Its Use in Treating Liver Stagnation in TCM"** by Chen and Chen (2004), *Chinese Medicine Journal*
A detailed look at how traditional Chinese herbs support liver detox.

24. **"Schisandra: An Herbal Approach to Liver Detoxification"** by Panossian et al. (2013), *Phytomedicine*
Discusses the hepatoprotective effects of schisandra.

25. **"Gut-Liver Axis: How the Microbiome Affects Detoxification"** by Zhang and Wang (2018), *Nature Reviews Gastroenterology & Hepatology*
Explores the relationship between gut health and liver detoxification.

26. **"Turmeric and Its Role in Liver Detox"** by Aggarwal et al. (2007), *Advances in Experimental Medicine and Biology*
Reviews curcumin's hepatoprotective and detoxifying properties.

27. **"The Role of Fasting in Enhancing Autophagy and Liver Detoxification"** by Levine et al. (2017), *Cell*
Discusses how fasting can boost liver detoxification through autophagy.

28. **"Milk Thistle and Its Role in Liver Regeneration"** by Abenavoli et al. (2010), *Journal of Clinical Gastroenterology*
Focuses on the protective and regenerative properties of milk thistle.

29. **"The Impact of Environmental Pollutants on Liver Health"** by Trasande et al. (2018), *Journal of Exposure Science and Environmental Epidemiology*
Explores how environmental toxins affect liver detox capacity.

30. **"Effects of Dietary Fibre on Liver Detoxification"** by Slavin (2013), *Journal of Nutrition*
Reviews the role of dietary fibre in supporting liver detox pathways.

Online Articles and Expert Blogs

31. **"How Liver Detoxification Works"** by Chris Kresser, *ChrisKresser.com*
An overview of how liver detox works and the best practices for supporting it.

32. **"Top Foods to Support Your Liver Detox"** by Dr. Mark Hyman, *DrHyman.com*
Discusses dietary interventions for liver detoxification.

33. **"What is Glutathione and Why Does Your Liver Need It?"** by Dr. Josh Axe, *DrAxe.com*
Focuses on the importance of glutathione in detox and how to boost it.

34. **"The Benefits of Intermittent Fasting for Liver Detox"** by Dr. Jason Fung, *DietDoctor.com*
Explores how intermittent fasting enhances liver detox processes.

35. **"Milk Thistle: A Natural Remedy for Liver Health"** by Andrew Weil, M.D., *DrWeil.com*
A comprehensive guide to milk thistle's liver-supportive properties.

36. **"How Toxins Impact Liver Function and How to Detoxify Safely"** by Dr. Amy Myers, *AmyMyersMD.com*
Provides strategies for reducing toxin load and supporting liver health.

37. **"Heavy Metal Detox: How to Safely Eliminate Toxins from Your Body"** by Dr. Edward Group, *Global Healing*
Reviews safe methods for detoxifying heavy metals.

38. **"Oligoscan Testing: A Modern Approach to Detecting Heavy Metal Toxicity"** by Dr. Lara Briden, *LaraBriden.com*
An explanation of how Oligoscan testing works and its role in detox plans.

39. **"Liver Detox Myths and Facts"** by The Cleveland Clinic
    A critical look at popular liver detox myths and the science behind real detox methods.

40. **"The Gut-Liver Connection: Why Your Gut Health Affects Liver Detox"** by Dr. Mercola, *Mercola.com*
    Discusses the gut-liver connection and how improving gut health boosts detox pathways.

Medical Websites and Health Organisations

41. **"Liver Disease and Detoxification"**, *American Liver Foundation*
    Provides information on how the liver detoxifies and strategies to prevent liver disease.

42. **"What You Should Know About Non-Alcoholic Fatty Liver Disease (NAFLD)"**, *Mayo Clinic*
    Offers a medical overview of NAFLD and its relationship to detoxification.

43. **"Glutathione and Its Role in Detoxification"**, *National Institutes of Health (NIH)*
    An in-depth look at glutathione and its importance in liver detox.

44. **"Milk Thistle and Liver Detox"**, *National Centre for Complementary and Integrative Health (NCCIH)*
    Reviews the scientific evidence supporting milk thistle's hepatoprotective effects.

45. "How the Liver Processes Toxins", *British Liver Trust*

www.ingramcontent.com/pod-product-compliance
Lightning Source LLC
Chambersburg PA
CBHW070032040426
42333CB00040B/1536